DR. MAYO'S BOY

A Century of American Medicine

Rob Tenery, MD

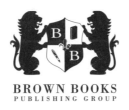

BROWN BOOKS
PUBLISHING GROUP

DR. MAYO'S BOY

For information, please contact:
Brown Books Publishing Group
16200 North Dallas Parkway, Suite 170
Dallas, Texas 75248
www.brownbooks.com
972-381-0009

A New Era in Publishing™

Paperback ISBN-13: 978-1-934812-24-2
Paperback ISBN-10: 1-934812-24-2

Hardbound ISBN-13: 978-1-934812-23-5
Hardbound ISBN-10: 1-934812-23-4

LCCN: 2008933967

1 2 3 4 5 6 7 8 9 10

DEDICATION

To Janet . . . who helped to develop this project from the start.
We have shared a lifetime of dreams together.

"The essence of what it means to be a physician, a true physician, is part science and part art. The science comes from medical school and continuing years of training. The art, that sense of conviction and compassion, comes from within and is learned at the bedside from patients and past physicians to whom this noble profession was more than their job. Medicine was their calling."

– Rob Tenery, MD

ACKNOWLEDGMENTS

To my mother, Barbara, who, at a time in my life when I lacked direction, never gave up on me. Her ability to fill in the gaps of my memory has made the stories in this book richer and fuller.

To David Groff who, as my first editor, took me under his wing and made me feel I really could become a part of the literary community. Through his mentoring, what at first was nothing more than a collection of recollections, we were able to craft a presentable manuscript.

To Milli, Kathryn, Janet, Latham, Michelle, Bill, Cathy, and Cindy at Brown Books Publishing, and Gene Blakeney, my son-in-law, whose collective expertise and vision allowed me to bring this book to fruition.

To my grandfather, Dr. W. C., who was steadfast in his belief that doctors' primary role was serving the needs of their patients. Always a leader, instead of talking about change, he made it happen.

Finally . . . to my father, Dr. Mayo. Even as he fought the ravages from his addiction to tobacco, his presence was never compromising. I still consider him the best physician I have ever seen. To pay him the ultimate compliment, he was not only my role model, he was my best friend.

CONTENTS

PART ONE

FOLLOWING HIS COATTAILS

PART TWO

MORE THAN THE MEDICINES

PART THREE

ON MY OWN

PART ONE

FOLLOWING HIS COATTAILS

1

HOUSE CALLS

I n 1948, there were only two surgeons in our small town. One was my grandfather, "Dr. W. C. Tenery." The other was his son and my father, known by everyone as "Dr. Mayo." In those days, all of our family activities revolved around the hospital and my father's obligations to his patients. If we went to the movies or out to eat, he let the hospital operator know exactly where he was. When my baby sister, Susie, and I spent time with both of our parents, the conversations often centered on my father's patients. If his patients were doing well, his mood was good and so was ours; if not, a pall fell over the family. My father had a tiring job, and he often dozed between bites of dinner. Despite the sacrifices, he was happy. More appropriately, he was satisfied, not so much from the money—he was occasionally paid in vegetables, loaves of bread, and homespun goods—but from the respect bestowed on him by his patients.

My introduction to calling on patients came when I was five. One evening my father pushed back from the dinner table, his meal only half-eaten. He glanced at me. "Do you want to make rounds?"

Even at five, I knew what he meant by "making rounds." Medicine was not only our life; it was our second language. This was the first time he'd asked me to join him. I looked up at my mother.

"Your tapioca will be here when you get back," she said.

I raced out the door behind him.

What I didn't realize then was that this night's excursion was the beginning of my lifelong journey into medicine—a discipline that, for physicians in my father's day, was more a calling than a job.

My father and I roared down the gravel road that formed a straight shot between our house and the hospital. Our home fronted Main Street, the major road through Waxahachie, but my father preferred the dusty back route. "Jefferson Street is more direct," he claimed often enough. With the medical emergencies my father and grandfather faced, seconds often made a difference.

Our community was a blend of country folk who lived off the land—mostly cotton and a little maize—and others who lived off those who lived off the land. To me, the good citizens of Waxahachie, Texas, were part of a giant, extended family. I didn't know all their names, but I recognized the faces. Big cities like Dallas, which was thirty miles to the north, seemed a million miles away. New York, where my mother's family lived, seemed planets away. Waxahachie's only real celebrity was Paul Richards, a former high school classmate of my father's and the manager of the Chicago White Sox. I'd met him only once and still beamed with pride when his name was broadcast over the radio.

"Why do you have to go back to the hospital?" I asked. "You were just there."

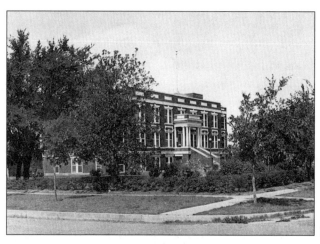

Waxahachie Sanitarium

"I guess a lot of nights, I don't have to," he said. "But it lets me sleep better if I do. Your grandfather feels the same. Now that I'm here, he has me do the checking for both of us. Kind of like your mother and I checking on you and your sister each night." The hospital stood in the far distance, its red-brick facade silhouetted in the dusky light. My father gave me a quick look. "Just stay by my side. If you have any questions, wait until we're back in the car."

The Men's Ward was a darkened room with rows of nondescript beds lining the walls. The beds were separated by off-white nightstands. I stayed close to my father, so close that the back of his jacket brushed my face. We stopped at the first bed. The nurse, Mrs. Delmer, scurried up to join us.

"Dr. Mayo, I didn't know you were here," she said.

He nodded.

"We had a little problem over in the emergency room just now. It's all taken care of." She straightened her starched nurse's hat, picked up the chart from the foot of the patient's bed, and started conversing with my father in a language I didn't understand. "Mr. Steed's temperature . . ."

My father pulled down Mr. Steed's bedsheets and stared at his chest.

After a few moments, we moved to the next bed. Mrs. Delmer scribbled notes on a piece of paper she kept tucked inside her breast pocket. She picked up the next chart, and my father repeated the procedure until we reached a bed in the far corner. The patient, a large man with a big stomach, was half asleep. My father glanced back at me, maybe to make sure I hadn't wandered off or maybe to make sure I had an eyeful of what was to come. He pulled down the sheet and began poking at a giant bandage crisscrossing the man's belly.

"Hey, Doc," the man said in a lazy voice. "Is that your boy?"

"It is. I thought I'd start him out early, see if he's cut out for this." His fingers worked their way to the far edge of the bandage. The man was huge; his naked stomach the size of an old leather, steamer trunk. To reach the far edge of the bandage, my father leaned over the man with both hands stretched out in front of him. "Maybe someday, he'll take over for me."

"You sure can be proud of your father," the man said. "If it wasn't for him, I wouldn't . . . ouch!" he screamed.

The man's squeal cut off his words and startled several patients. I heard a collective groan coming from the room. The bloodstained bandage was clasped in my father's hand.

"That didn't hurt me at all," he said and handed the soiled dressing to Mrs. Delmer.

"Thanks Doc," the man said. "I knew that was coming. I just didn't know when."

"Mrs. Delmer will put on a fresh bandage, only this one will be smaller." He turned to me. "Sometimes you have to go through a little hurt before things get better."

When my father invited me to watch my first surgery, I couldn't have been more excited. He stood at the scrub sink, his arms covered with soap up to his elbows. He backed away and peered into the operating room where my grandfather stood atop a small step stool overlooking his patient. My grandfather was a small man, closer to my size than most adults, but his presence made him appear to tower above others around him. He glanced at my father and then at me.

"Is he going to help?"

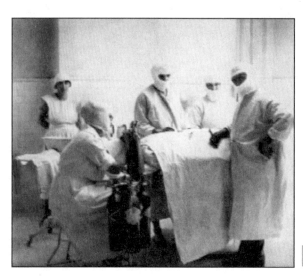

Dr. W. C. standing to the right in the operating room

"Since he made rounds with me," my father said, "I thought he ought to see what we do in here."

"Just so long as he doesn't get in the way."

My grandfather, Dr. W. C., as his patients called him, was all business when it came to his hospital. He'd have no favorites, not even his only grandson. He'd come to Texas from the hills of Tennessee in the back of a covered wagon. He had started this very hospital in a converted rooming house almost thirty-five years ago. Later, when the old structure wasn't big enough, he helped the town raise bonds to pay for the new building.

When I thought about it, I wasn't sure I wanted to be there. If my father hadn't insisted, I'd have gladly traded in my oversized white pajamas and the cap and mask for my old blue-jeans and a T-shirt.

"He'll be fine," my father said. He nudged me into the tile-covered room with his knee. He reached for a towel from the nurse and carefully wiped the water from his hands and arms, then slung the towel in the direction of a basket in the far corner. To me, he said, "You stand up there by Miss Jones. Use the stool, so you can see."

"Come on over here," Miss Jones said.

Oma Jones was our nurse anesthetist. Like my grandfather, she was legendary in our community, not so much for what she did, but for what she didn't do. She refused to put a patient to sleep until she was good and ready. Oma had a great deal of control, often delaying surgery for hours until she finished her plans. Her career was her life. She owned a parrot, Ben, who, according to my father, was the only object of her affection.

"You're not going to pass out on me are you?" Miss Jones said. "I can only take care of one patient at a time."

Until then, fainting hadn't crossed my mind. As I crawled onto the stool, I felt everyone watching. "There," I said, proud that I'd settled in. The pungent smell of ether and my own hot breath under my mask made breathing difficult. My grandfather nodded to my father. The surgery was about to begin.

My father took a scalpel in his gloved hand. The metal blade glistened under the intense light. In one quick thrust, he buried the blade into the patient's abdomen and opened up a wide gash that ran down past the belly button. Blood and fat erupted like lava. At exactly that moment, a wave of nausea welled up in my throat. My fingers groped for a better hold on my stool. The blood and the smells and the dizziness were too much for a kid who hadn't asked for any of this. I held my ground for less than a minute and then toppled from the stool. I hit the tile floor head first. In the far distance, I heard Oma Jones say, "Future doctors *never* faint."

* ■ ■

A week after my nosedive from the stool, my blackened eye had faded. In a strange way, I felt I'd accomplished something. Now, more than ever, I wanted to be a doctor. Working my way back into the operating room, well, that would take time. Down the long hallway, I could hear my mother trying to quiet my baby sister. Counting Susie, our family had grown to six, if you included our two dogs. I waited eagerly by the back door. My father sipped the last of his after-dinner coffee and prepared to leave.

"Not this time," he said. He waved me aside, pulled open the screen door, and moved into the doorway. "Your mother's still upset with me over your black eye."

"My eye's okay. It's almost pink again in parts. Look here—"

"It's not only that."

"Then why?"

"Because this time it's different," he said. "I'm going to make rounds at the other hospital."

"What other hospital?"

"Maybe when you're a little older." My father let the screen door bang closed behind him.

I swung open the door and ran after him. I caught the tail of his jacket. "Please."

He stopped and looked off into the distance for a long moment, and then nodded. I poked my head back in the door to tell my mother and dashed out to the car all before she could respond.

We pulled out on Main Street and didn't take the dusty shortcut down Jefferson. Instead, we headed in the opposite direction. I looked in the backseat and noticed the black doctor's bag, the one my father rarely used.

"What's that for?"

"The hospital where we're going, they don't have much. Besides, we're also going to make a house call." He smiled. "She and her family have been friends of ours for as long as I can remember."

I sat back against the warm velour seat.

My father gave up only small bits of information at a time. I'd gotten all I was going to get. The large Victorian homes of our neighbors glowed as we got closer to the Square. We passed Waxahachie's grandiose, red-granite courthouse with its stunning clock tower, tall enough to be seen from ten miles away. Our courthouse was famous around Texas, partly for its size and beauty and partly for the dozen or more faces carved into the four porch capitals. Some of the stone faces were beautiful, others were grotesque. Legend has it a German stone carver fell in love with a local girl. At first, he cast her with full cheeks and a bashful smile. But, the myth says, when she didn't return his love, he carved new versions with long, demon-like faces and a grimacing mouth of fangs or missing teeth.

Except for the marquee at the entrance to the Texas Theater, the rest of downtown was closed up tight. My father pressed on the accelerator and we continued east into a part of town I knew little about. The street signs still read Main, but to me it looked as if we'd moved backward in time. Our side of town had streetlights; this side did not. The houses had shrunk to paint-worn structures no larger than our garage. I saw shadows of people in the windows preparing to bed down for the night. Many of the yards were bald patches of dirt. A smoky fog hung to the ground and the scent of burning logs trickled through our car window. Despite the unfamiliar surroundings, I wasn't afraid.

A good mile or so past the courthouse, we pulled to a stop in front of a small white frame house. This was a part of town my father called Freeman, populated mostly by Negroes who worked for people on our side of town.

"Come on in and meet Ollie," he said, reaching for his bag in the backseat.

As we made our way up the walkway, I noticed the worn clapboard on the house, its paint peeling, the boards close to the ground rotted in long uneven sections. Side-stepping a big hole in the concrete, I ducked under my father's outstretched arm as he held open the screen door. Then I saw Ollie, her wide, ivory eyes and chocolate face atop the largest body I had ever seen.

"Docta' Mayo," she called out. "Is dat your boy? He sure is cute, kind of resembles Miz Barbara." She reached out and gave me a pat on my cheeks.

"Ollie, I need to check your blood pressure." He opened up his bag, bent down, and fumbled to get the elastic cuff wrapped around her large arm.

"I try so hard to lose some weight." She held her arm. "But those pies. I just can't help myself. You knows how good they is. I remembers when I made one for you when you was just a little boy. If I recalls, you nearly ate the whole thing—"

"Shhh." He pumped air into the cuff. He repeated the procedure several times before he let the air slip out. "Ollie, with blood pressure as high as yours, you should have been dead twenty years ago. You been taking your medicine?"

"I always does what you tells me. Except for the pies."

He handed her a handful of pills, samples he'd extracted from his bag. "This should hold you until I get back next week."

Ollie scooped up the samples, then struggled to get to her feet. "Let me send you home some of my coconut custard pie for Miz Barbara and your boy here. You knows how she likes it too."

My father made no attempt to resist her offer, and Ollie disappeared into the depths of her tiny home. She returned with several slices of pie wrapped in wax paper. In her free hand, she clutched two wrinkled one-dollar bills. "This is all I have for now, but I'll get you more when I can."

"The pie is payment enough." He grabbed his bag and nudged open the tattered screen door with his shoulder. "See you next week."

When we were back in the car, I asked, "Why didn't you take the money?"

"When I was about your age, Ollie worked for our family. I'm just doing what I can to pay her back."

We had gone only four blocks when we pulled over. We were in the middle of downtown Freeman in front of the Cotton Club. The facade was old and paint peeled from the siding. Unfamiliar music rumbled out into the darkened street. Hunkering down in my seat, I began to rethink my decision to come along.

"It's not what it seems," my father said. "At least, not exactly."

Out of the shadows, a very large man with dark skin walked up and tapped on the window.

"I'll watch the car for you, Doc." His voice was firm. "Ain't nobody going to lay a hand on it, not while I's around."

My father nodded, then turned and grabbed his bag from the backseat. "Let's go, but you stay close to me." My father looked back at the man now leaning against the trunk. "Is your wife still doing okay, Cleveland?"

The man gave him a wide smile. "That she is. Thank you for askin'."

My father swung open the door, and we disappeared inside the Cotton Club.

The acrid fumes of tobacco smoke stung my nose. In the dim light in the far corner, I recognized a jukebox vibrating with the unfamiliar sounds. People lined the wall, which were plastered with faded movie posters. A few people danced in the center of the room.

"I'm sure glad you're here, Dr. Mayo," a lady said. Her voice broke in from somewhere off to the side. Her skin was brown like Ollie's. She wore white nurse's shoes, skirt, and cap with a red-sequined blouse.

"It's Theta Sims, Dr. Mayo. She ain't doing so good."

"Let's take a look, Priscilla. I brought more penicillin." He moved quickly through the club to the back.

Priscilla stopped and looked at me. "Is this your boy? If he's anything like you and Dr. W. C., he's sure gonna make a fine doctor some day."

Embarrassed, I drew away at her attention to me. I followed my father's coattails as he slid back a curtain and entered a room at the rear of the building. Beds lined the walls, nearly all of them filled with sweaty, groaning people.

"I moved her over there, so I could be near," Priscilla said. "Besides, she'll be closer to the fan and you knows how hot it gets back here sometimes."

A single bulb hung from an exposed cord in the middle of the ceiling. There was a small lamp on Priscilla's desk. Beds lined the walls, and the pungent, medicinal smell floating around the room reminded me of the hospital on our side of town. The similarities ended there. Male and female patients, along with a few kids close to my age, lay on beds of every shape and configuration. Wooden vegetable crates covered with cloth served as bedside stands.

I hung back by the door. My father set his bag on Priscilla's desk and moved over to examine a patient.

"I'll bet you never met a nurse like me," Priscilla said. She edged closer to me. I knew she was trying to make me feel more comfortable while we waited for my father. "This is my place. I cover both sides, the club and the hospital. One minute I'm a hostess, the next a nurse. My people got no other choice. I'm all they have."

My father straightened and motioned for Priscilla to join him.

"The penicillin isn't going to be enough," he said. "Looks like a ruptured appendix. We'll have to operate tonight. Get the ambulance and meet me at the hospital in about an hour."

He moved from patient to patient, talking mostly and handing out a few samples from his bag. My father reassured each that he'd do what he could. After a while, he closed his bag and headed for the door where I was waiting. There was no need to signal. I was two steps ahead of him.

"Thanks, Cleveland," my father said to the man safeguarding our car. We pulled away and headed toward our side of town. We didn't talk much for the first part of the trip home.

"Why are those people in the Cotton Club and not in the hospital?" I asked.

"If they were, the people on our side of town wouldn't come to the hospital when they got sick. They'd go to Dallas instead." He peered at me and said, "If you're going to become a doctor, you have to be color-blind."

2

A Walk in Their Footsteps

I wasn't sure I was cut out to be a doctor. After years of watching my father and grandfather push their weary bodies past exhaustion when patients needed them, I'd come to view them as quasi-mythical figures. I could never walk in their shoes. I sensed that my mother, who paid the highest price for my father's commitment to his patients, seemed relieved that I didn't ache to be a doctor.

In the summer of 1954, just two weeks after completion of the seventh grade at Marvin Elementary, my parents cut off my allowance. The idea was to instill in me a sense of responsibility. I felt it was cruel and unusual punishment.

I needed money for the summer and I had only two options—hire on as a sacker at Wyatt's grocery or work as an orderly at the hospital. Neither job thrilled me. The pay was the same—fifty cents an hour. The hospital included meals. Though hospital food was a small step above the school cafeteria, a free lunch was still a free lunch.

I took the job at the hospital and began sooner than I expected.

I stood in the corner of our small kitchen, my head in the refrigerator.

My father was on the phone speaking to the caller in his reassuring doctor's voice. "I understand. We'll be right there." He hung up the phone and looked over at me, his eyes troubled. "You don't officially start until morning, but I need you now. Let's go."

I couldn't imagine what calamity awaited us at the other end of Jefferson Street.

After a quick peck on my mother's cheek and a nod to my baby sister who was already fast asleep, my father headed for the door. We jumped into the car, sped down the driveway, and turned onto the dusty road.

"You may not like what you're about to see," he said, "but if you're going to be a doctor, there's one thing you must learn—you never walk away."

Pushing down on the accelerator, we raced over the old railway crossing that marked the halfway point to the hospital. The old car's shocks groaned.

At the hospital, two ambulances, their lights ablaze, and two Highway Patrol cars were parked outside the emergency room doors.

"What's going on?" I asked.

"There's been an accident. No, that's not true. It was not an accident."

He pulled into the only remaining slot in the parking area.

A uniformed Highway Patrol officer stood by the emergency room. "It's a bad one, Doc. She took a blast to the head. I don't know how, but she's still holding on."

"Anyone else?"

"The father was gone when we got there. The justice of the peace pronounced him dead at the scene."

"What about the child?" my father asked.

"What kind of animal shoots a ten-month-old? Middle of the back. He was alive when we brought him in."

Chaos reigned in the emergency room. My father disappeared into the crowd. Unfamiliar people scurried in and out of the doors. I peered around their backs and legs, trying to see what was going on. I saw a gurney tucked away in the corner. Face down on the gurney lay the infant the officer had been talking about. The baby whimpered and I realized that no one was attending to him.

A hand touched my shoulder. "Your father needs you," Mrs. Delmer said.

"What about the baby?"

"Your father checked on him. He had to make a choice." She drew in a deep breath. "Now, go on in and help your father."

I held back my tears as she gently pulled the sheet up over the child's body.

I shoved my way through the crowd into the operating arena of the emergency room and found my father. For the moment, he was the only thing that made sense.

His gloved hands were soaked in blood. "How about you help pump?"

I crawled up on a stool and got my first glance of the young woman, the baby's mother. She had smooth brown skin and matted, blood-soaked hair. Blood was being transfused into her body through tubes in each arm and one leg. Large red bottles of blood hung on stands at the foot of the table. My father was focused. He handed the nurse one bloody instrument after another, only to have it replaced by a clean one.

"Here," a nurse said to me. "You pump in the rest of this unit, while I run over to the lab and get what's left."

After a few minutes of pumping, my hands ached.

My father moved away from the table and stripped off his gloves. Half the woman's face and neck was blown away.

"You can stop," he said to me.

Mrs. Delmer pulled a sheet out of the cabinet and draped it over the baby's mother.

"What about the baby?" my father asked.

She shook her head.

The Highway Patrol officer stood at the door of the operating arena. My father asked, "What caused all this?"

"When she could talk, the mother said the family stopped to get gas at a station in Italy. She asked how much for a Dr Pepper. The gas jockey told them two bucks a bottle for a fifteen cent soda. She said something and the son-of-a-bitch pulled out a twelve gauge. He emptied it into their car."

"This guy, you have him in custody?"

"We have him. He didn't even try to run. He's white, she's a Negro. You know how juries are. He'll probably be out in three, five max." He turned toward the body on the operating table. "If things happened the other way around, there wouldn't be enough police officers in Ellis County to keep them from hanging the bastard."

My father shook his head and slowly turned away.

On the ride home, I asked, "Why did he shoot those people?"

My father pulled into our driveway and brought the car to a stop. "Fear and prejudice and stupidity."

The next morning, I leaned against the gurney and waited for my first assignment.

"Do whatever Willie says," my grandfather had told me earlier.

I'd known Willie for as long as I could remember. He was a towering figure with a permanent smile. I was told his smile didn't falter even when his wife nearly died giving birth to their oldest. Willie, along with two other men, Leon and Jo-Jo, made up the transportation team at the hospital.

I saw them more as patient movers than anything else.

"Dr. W. C. has a way with words, don't he?" Willie said, "Let's you and me check by surgery to see who needs a ride."

Lanita Hawthorne, the head nurse, said, "Willie, they need you in 205. It's Veda Sneed. She's not going to surgery unless you take her."

Miss Veda, as folks called her, was the matriarch of Waxahachie society and owner of our meager claims to culture—three movie theaters, a drive-in, and the Chautauqua Auditorium, where the only official function still held there was the annual high school graduation ceremony. When she was in the hospital, everyone catered to her— everyone except Lanita Hawthorne, who stayed out of her way.

Willie pushed through the door to 205, and I followed right behind. An empty gurney sat beside her bed. Miss Sneed was railing at Leon and Jo-Jo, who cowered in the far corner behind a giant wicker armchair.

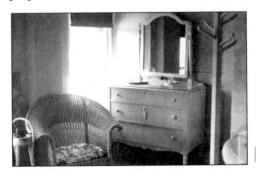

Patient room at the hospital

"Miss Veda," Willie said, his ever-present smile turned up two hundred watts. "Where do you want me to take you this fine day, all dressed up in your bright yellow bathrobe?"

"I was supposed to be in surgery. I'd been there too, if someone hadn't sent these replacements."

"They're not replacements, Miss Veda. We're part of the same team. Now why don't you slide over here on the gurney, so we can get you to surgery?"

And with that, we conveyed Miss Veda to the operating room.

A week later, Jo-Jo and I rushed a patient and gurney to the operating room. We were late, and we'd gotten a bit reckless with our speed and direction. In the hallway up ahead, my grandfather walked toward us. He dragged behind him a skeleton on wheels.

"What are you doing, Pa?" I asked, hoping to deflect his attention from our runaway gurney.

He looked up just in time to avoid a collision. "Oh," he blurted out. "I'm taking George here over to give our nursing students an anatomy lesson." He rattled the makeshift contraption.

The gurney bounced off a wall. I glanced back over my shoulder where the patient continued to snooze. Jo-Jo, on the other hand, had vanished. I brought the stretcher to a full stop not five feet from the operating room. Pa laughed for several long moments.

"What's so funny?" I asked.

"George, here," he said, pointing at the skeleton, "and Jo-Jo don't get along."

"Why is that? It's just a collection of old bones."

"Not to Jo-Jo. His parents came from Haiti. He believes in voodoo. He and his family believe a human bone is possessed by evil spirits unless it's been cleansed by a medicine man."

"You're a doctor. Can't you do that?"

"Not as far as Jo-Jo is concerned. Last year, when his son got sick, he refused to bring him to see me. Instead, he took him to a medicine man out in the country." His smile faded. "As you grow up, you're going to find out there are many different types of doctors in this world."

"Quacks, you mean?"

My grandfather pushed George against the wall and walked up to the stretcher to examine my patient. "Some are and some aren't. A good doctor never has all the answers. The best are those who aren't afraid to admit it."

———— ■ ■ ————

As the Texas sun beat down on the gravel parking lot behind the hospital, my father checked the bandage he had just applied to a patient's abdomen. Certain it was secure, he patted Sam on the shoulder.

"Sam, remember what I said about giving this time to heal. I already checked with Tucker and told him you wouldn't be back to work at the gas station for awhile. Three weeks or so. We don't want that hernia to open up on you." He was reluctant to send his patient back to the Cotton Club so soon after surgery. "Priscilla will change your dressing in the morning. I'll be over to check on you tomorrow night."

"Thanks, Docta' Mayo, for what-all you done for me."

Two attendants from Blum-Marshall Funeral Home scooped Sam up on the stretcher and headed for the ambulance.

"I likes to work, and my family sure could use the money," Sam said, "but if that's what you tell me."

My father called to Buddy. "Make sure you and Mike don't jostle him and mess up my good work."

"You know me, Doc," Buddy said. "Only the best for your patients. We'll handle him like a china tea service. If you want, we'll take your boy there along to check us out and bring him right back."

I hoped my father would say I could go. I'd always had a fascination with ambulances. I'd only ridden in one once. That was when Mr. Blum asked me along for the Homecoming parade.

"Please," I said to my father. "Willie says we're finished for the day."

"Just drive slowly," he said to Buddy, then caught my sleeve. "Maybe in your day, things will be different and we won't have morticians delivering patients to backroom hospitals."

I scooted into the front seat between Buddy and Mike, then waved goodbye to my father. Soon the ambulance reached No-Man's Land— that dusty-brown stretch of road outside the Square, but not yet in Freeman—a place where straggly blades of Johnson grass dotted the cracked ground. The engine abruptly choked and coughed. Buddy scanned the gauges for a problem and turned toward Mike for an answer. Nothing. After limping along another hundred feet or so, the ambulance shut down. Buddy let it coast silently to the side of the road.

"I'll be damned," Buddy said. He eased out of the ambulance and ambled to the front of the vehicle, where Mike had already popped the hood.

I slipped out and peered around Buddy's wide stomach.

"What do you think?" Buddy asked, his giant gut pressed up against the hot fender.

"Hell, I don't know," Mike said. "All I do is put gas in these sons-a-bitches."

We stood there for fifteen minutes staring at each other. I drew circles in the dirt with the toe of my shoe.

"Why don't you let me take a look?" Sam asked. Buddy spun around, his eyes widening as he came face-to-face with Sam. He was wrapped in a sheet.

"You know what Doc said," Buddy answered, his voice uneasy. "And with his boy here, he'd have our butts if he saw you out here like this."

"How else we going to get this fixed and me on to Priscilla's to get some rest?"

Buddy looked up and down the deserted road, then back over at the two of us. With the square a hundred yards back up the road and Freeman off in the distance, he nodded in frustration.

Sam worked under the hood for a good ten minutes. With the late afternoon sun beating down, I sought relief inside the ambulance. "Give it a try," he said.

Buddy jumped back in the ambulance. A quick turn on the ignition, and the motor purred back to life. "Get in," he said. "We've got to get you to Priscilla's."

Wincing, Sam looked at his bandage—no signs of blood and everything still intact. He limped to the rear of the ambulance and slowly climbed in.

3

MY FIRST PATIENT

———■·——

I graduated from Marvin Elementary and looked forward to starting my freshman year of high school. Again, I had to find employment for the summer. My father lured me back to the hospital by offering me a job as assistant technician in the laboratory. With the new job came a pay raise to seventy-five cents an hour. My title was assistant technician, but in truth I was head urine tester and general flunky. Lab work was a lousy job by most accounts. The lab smelled of stale urine. I was short, and the containers stacked on the counter were never far from my sensitive nose.

"There's more in the refrigerator," Lenny Pope said. "Must have been left over from yesterday's late shift."

"Thanks," I said.

Aside from the smells, the laboratory resembled most other areas of the hospital—the same off-white walls with cabinets and shelves filled with boxes that reached to the ceiling. Except for the specimens strewn across the counters, everything had its place. The lab had a centrifuge in the corner, two microscopes that were off limits to me, a large refrigerator, and a row of animal cages in the back room.

My job was to calculate the volume of liquid in each jar, rate each for clarity, and test for protein, sugar, blood, and pH. I made one final test for specific gravity and passed the smelly liquid to Lenny for a microscopic analysis. Watching the mercury-filled thermometer bob up and down in a sea of urine was the only part of the process I enjoyed. My father's suggestion that I get to know the medical business from the bottom up struck me as too literal. Then again, at seventy-five cents an hour, meals included, I wasn't in a position to complain.

"Don't forget to feed Connie and the others," Lenny said. "Remember, tomorrow will be her last supper." He made a slashing motion across his neck.

That was the other part of my new assignment—keeper of laboratory animals—specifically, the rabbits used to determine whether female patients were pregnant. How it worked was, the patient's urine was injected into the rabbit. If the patient was pregnant, a hormone in her urine caused a change in the rabbit's ovaries. To get the results, the rabbit had to be dissected and its ovaries examined. Even at thirteen, I was struck by the irony of animals giving up their lives to determine if someone else was creating a new one. If the patient was an unwed mother, that new life would likely be snuffed out before it started.

My father and grandfather did not terminate pregnancies. The names of those who did, including one of our town's physicians, were well known in the community. From what I could glean from my boss, Lenny Pope, the abortions took place after hours in a dingy back room of the doctor's office. He claimed all it took was saline, a coat hanger, and a rubber hose. Lenny left the rest of the grisly details to my imagination. Talk of abortion never took place openly, or it was discussed in the open only because my father or grandfather was called in to save the life of a young girl dying from complications of a botched abortion.

"I'll feed them as soon as I get through with these," I said. I glanced back at the row of putrid smelling jars.

I liked the rabbits, especially Connie with her one floppy ear. I'd informally made her a mascot of the laboratory, frequently letting her run free. Lenny didn't approve. He never said anything, but I could tell he wasn't happy putting up with the Doc's kid. He said it was by chance that nine days earlier he'd pulled Connie from her cage and injected her. I think it was Lenny's way of showing me who was boss.

In the days since, I had formulated a plan to get Connie a reprieve. I would plead her case to my father.

I'd hurried through the rest of my day's work, hoping to catch my father before we headed home for dinner. I was always more likely to get my way when it was just the two of us. Right now, Connie and I could use every advantage. I scuttled through the door to his office. He walked out of his small bathroom adjacent to the office. Behind him trailed a plume of cigarette smoke. I thought about asking him if he'd really quit, as he had promised my mother, and decided against it.

"I want a pet," I said.

"You want what?" He settled into his chair behind a stack of medical files that blocked my view of him.

"It's my birthday on the twenty-fourth. I want a pet," I answered. "I'll take care of her. You and mother won't have to do anything."

"You said *her*."

"It's Connie, one of the rabbits over in the laboratory. She's the one with the floppy ear."

"As long as your mother gives her okay. And Lenny is willing to let her go."

"That may be a problem," I said. "Lenny needs to . . ." I searched for the right words.

"What does a rabbit cost? Three, maybe five dollars at the most. He must have a dozen over there already. If he complains, tell him I'll pay for it."

I stared blankly at my father.

"Don't tell me this rabbit of yours has already been injected." He gave me a cautious look, sliding the pile of charts to the side. "Well, has it?"

"Ten days ago tomorrow."

"Then you better find another pet." My father rocked back in his chair. "Unless Weedon or Kelly are willing to help."

My father was referring to the two veterinarians in town. "Kelly is on vacation and Weedon is backed up. His nurse said he couldn't get to it until the end of the week, if then." I could feel my pulse quicken. "You're a surgeon; rabbits can't be that much different than people. Back in medical school, didn't you tell me you worked in a research lab that used rabbits? All you have to do is open her up, look at her ovaries, then sew her back up. I'll nurse her back to health."

"It's not that simple," he said.

"Lenny Pope does it all the time, and he's just a lab technician." Comparing my father's surgical skills to a man twenty years his junior with only two years of college was cruel, but I was desperate.

"I don't have any idea how much anesthetic to give an animal."

"Weedon's nurse said just put some gauze over her nose and drip ether over it until she doesn't flinch when you pinch her. Maybe you can talk Oma Jones into helping. After all, with that parrot of hers, maybe she has a soft spot for animals." I knew it was a long-shot. "You could tell her it's for my birthday."

He said he'd think about it, but I knew he'd already made up his mind.

Relieved that my father would see things my way with Connie, I worked with extra zeal. I scurried around the nurses' station, my tray overloaded with tubes of blood and jars of urine, before making my way back to the lab.

"Here, Robbie." Mrs. Delmer put a beaker of urine onto the pile. "Old Mr. Potter takes all morning to collect a specimen. He really ought to get his prostate reamed out while your father is removing his gallbladder. The old geezer won't give up. All that blather about the sanctity of his private parts." She grinned at me. "I've seen them, and between you and me, he's carrying nothing special down there."

I tried to force a grin, covering up my embarrassment. "I've got to get these back over to the lab," I said.

"You know, I've never understood why some people put so much importance on the smallest things." She broke into a laugh and quickly choked it off. "Good morning, Dr. W. C."

My grandfather uttered no more than a grunt before disappearing into the room across the hall.

I made it to the end of the hall, when I heard an ominous gagging sound. I stopped, nudging the door to room 210 with my shoulder. I saw a patient covered in vomit. She was writhing in the bed. I jumped back, tipping over several of the jars, set down the tray, and dashed back to the nurses' station. "Mrs. Delmer! Pa! There's a . . ."

Mrs. Delmer's face appeared in the doorway, followed by my grandfather's. "There's a lady!" I was barely able to cough out. "Down in 210. I think she's having a seizure!"

Mrs. Delmer sped past me.

My grandfather trailed close behind. "Who is it?"

Mrs. Delmer looked back. "It's Mildred Easton. She's Dr. Dyess' patient. She's supposed to have twins next week. He put her in the hospital to control her blood pressure."

I inched my way down the hall to recapture my tray and assess the damage. Mrs. Delmer's head burst out of the door in my direction. "Run to surgery and get the Lap Pac, now!"

The Lap Pac was a special set of instruments set aside for unexpected surgical emergencies outside of the operating room. She disappeared back into the patient's room. I grabbed the Lap Pac from surgical supply, cloaked in the sterile outer covering and rushed back to 210.

"Here," I called out.

"Wait in the hall. We might need you to do something else." Mrs. Delmer turned back toward the patient's bed.

I peeked around her, catching only a glimpse of my grandfather, stethoscope in his ears, hunched over the still patient.

In the hall, I picked up my tray. Three bottles of urine had spilled. One of them belonged to old man Potter. I hoped Mrs. Delmer would spare me from telling him he'd have to come up with another specimen. Minutes later, the door to 210 opened and my grandfather eased into the hall. In his hands, he held a small baby hidden by a bloody sheet. "Thanks," he said, looking across at me. "He wouldn't have made it, if it wasn't for you." He cradled the crying infant. "I've got to get him over to the nursery."

Mrs. Delmer stepped into the doorway, her ivory white starched uniform spattered with red blood. "Ask Leon and Willie to come," she said. "Your grandfather saved one of the babies."

"What about Mrs. Easton?"

"I'm afraid not." Mrs. Delmer looked away, as a tear rolled down her cheek. "Sometimes you think you've seen it all. You think none of it can bother you. Then you realize you're wrong."

The next day, after trying to satisfy nearly every doctor in the hospital, I finally made it to the waiting room off the operating room suite. My father agreed to operate on Connie, but only after all his other obligations had been completed. And they had started without me.

I stopped by the nursery to check on the baby boy my grandfather delivered the day before. Mrs. Delmer had the same idea. She held the infant in her hands, pressing his little cheek to hers. "Want to hold him?" she asked.

At first, I felt reluctant, since my only experience holding babies was with my younger sister a long time ago. To me, all babies looked the same. Some were darker, some lighter. But when she laid his little body in my arms, he seemed different. I wrapped my hand around his head. He would never know his mother or his twin brother.

He puckered his lips.

"He's rooting for his mother," Mrs. Delmer told me, then pressed a nippled bottle in my hand.

The baby latched onto the nipple. Here I was, rescuing a three-dollar lab rabbit from Lenny Pope, and I couldn't do more to save this baby's mother.

"If I'd only gone by Mrs. Easton's room sooner," I said.

"What if you hadn't gone by at all?" She gently lifted the baby out of my arms and laid him back in the bassinet. "Isn't your rabbit about to have surgery?"

"Yeah, I've got to go." I arrived as the door to the operating suite swung open. "Is she . . . ?" I called out, expecting to see my father. But it was only Rita Marvin, the circulating nurse. She quickly disappeared into the sterile supply closet without so much as a glance. I knew she was mad at me. In fact, they all were, especially Oma Jones, who'd agreed to help only after my father promised her his two behind-the-dugout seats at an upcoming Chicago White Sox exhibition game in Dallas. I was the only one at the hospital who put much value in a floppy-eared rabbit. I had been assigned to be Connie's keeper, but somewhere along the way, I'd become her protector too.

I waited for Rita Marvin to emerge from the closet then stepped squarely in her path. "How's Connie doing?"

"The rabbit is doing fine." She glanced at her wristwatch. "That rabbit's surgery has delayed my dinner. What I don't understand is why you care so much about a damned rabbit."

"Because, Miss Marvin, that rabbit happens to be my first patient."

4

THEY PAID WHAT THEY COULD

After the episode with Connie, I needed a change of venue. Six weeks of testing noxious body fluids and cleaning up animal excrement was enough. Either I'd move to another area at the hospital or I'd tie on a sacker's apron at Wyatt's grocery. Under the pretext that I wanted a broader exposure to the medical field, I got my father to transfer me to radiology for the rest of summer. Mostly I worked in the darkroom, loading and unloading X-ray cassettes, then drying and cropping the films before they were placed in the patients' files.

I dropped in on Lenny Pope unannounced. "I see things don't change much around here."

"How's that rabbit of yours?" he asked, looking up from his battered microscope.

"Connie, she's fine," I said. "Had to move her to a cage in the backyard after she kept chewing through the telephone cords. My father threatens to take her out to the Jarratt's farm, but so far, she's still at home." The truth was that Connie's frequent bowel movements and her habit of gnawing on anything in her reach turned out to be a lot more trouble than I expected. Not willing to admit my mistake, I secretly hoped my father would make good on his threat.

Lenny scribbled a note on one of the lab sheets, slid the glass slide out from under the microscope, and replaced it with another.

"In one of my periodicals, I read about a test for pregnancy where we won't need rabbits." He glanced back at the row of cages that lined the far wall. "It never set right with me anyway. Killing those animals just to see if some high-school sweetheart was messing around."

After spending half the summer working together, this was a side of Lenny Pope I hadn't seen. I realized that Lenny and my father had at least one thing in common: it had to do with preserving life.

There wasn't a cloud in the sky that Sunday afternoon my father invited me to go out shooting. He had an old .22 lever-action he kept in the hall closet. He wasn't much of an outdoorsman, so when he offered, I jumped.

"You bet," I said. His days were so consumed with his patients that I was proud he was willing to spend time with me outside of the hospital.

We drove over to a field on old man Martin's farm. We'd been there once, four years before, when he first purchased the gun. The field was far enough out of the way that any errant bullets wouldn't hit anything. We pulled to a stop under one of the giant pecan trees. "Native," he called the old trees. "Hulls so thick they're no good for shelling, but the trees do make a good shade." I tumbled out of the car, eager to get away from the stink inside. My father filled his socks with chunks of the bright yellow sulfur powder to ward off chiggers. Me, I'd rather put up with the irritating bites. My father would not.

"You set up some cans, while I load the gun," he said. He handed me a paper sack full of empty Campbell's bean cans, a staple at our house.

"What about we do some hunting instead?"

"Never got into that," he said. He loaded shells into the gun's cartridge. "Not that I'm critical of those who do. It just seems like a contradiction for me to devote my career to saving lives and then spend my free time killing defenseless animals."

The time we spent together, just the two of us, like that day on old man Martin's farm, were rare. I saw him often enough at home and in passing at the hospital, but the minutes we spent alone never seemed long enough.

I often arrived at the radiology lab early. I'd pull the morning's X-rays out of the fixer and hang the film on the rack to dry.

One morning, Ruby Profett and I huddled together in the small alcove that housed the X-ray machine and fluoroscopy unit. Ruby was a radiology technician and my current boss. She was well into her seventies, and she'd worked at the hospital since long before I was born. She had flaming red hair out of a bottle that you could spot a mile away.

"What's that bulldozer doing out back?" I asked.

"I've heard rumors, but you know how they are. Your grandfather has his lips sealed on this one. I heard when he presented his plan to the board, a couple of them threw a fit. He told them he'd put up a building on his own and move his practice into it if they refused to go along. That calmed them down."

The door to the X-ray room swung open. Willie said, "The ambulance just brought in a bad car accident. They need the portable machine over in the emergency room, STAT!"

In the late 1940s, our community was called the Cotton Capital of the World. Waxahachie was on a major highway, dead-center of cotton country. Two railroad lines cut through town, and we were close to a number of gins. The result was a fair number of major emergencies. I hung up the last film and dashed out the door tugging on the portable X-ray machine.

"You take the back and I'll get the front," Ruby said.

I stepped around to the rear of the cart. Ruby wrapped her hands around its long, upstretched neck and we pushed and pulled the monster to the emergency room. We rounded the corner and saw a horde of people jammed in the hallway.

"Let us through," Ruby called out.

"Over there," my father said, pointing a bloody, gloved finger at a patient on the operating table. "Get a skull series and an AP of her chest." He turned back to another patient lying on an ambulance gurney.

Ruby deftly tilted the patient up and slid the film cassette under her back. "You'll be okay," she whispered in the patient's ear.

"What about my husband?" the woman asked. "Is he going to be okay?"

"Please be still, dearie. The doctor is with him now. This will only take a minute."

I struggled to position the neck of the machine directly over the patient's chest.

"Get the apron," Ruby said.

The apron was a fifteen-pound, lead-lined shield worn by people like Ruby and me who took the X-rays. I was engulfed as I draped the heavy garment around my neck and body. "Where do you want me?"

"Hold the cassette, there." Ruby turned and shouted, "Everybody out."

A couple of nurses and a technician scurried from the room to avoid the radiation. I could hear the machine warming up, and then the noise rose to a high whine before going quiet again.

After taking two headshots while I held the film cassette in the proper position, Ruby waved everyone back into the room. She rushed back to radiology to develop the film.

My father examined the blood-stained face of the man lying on the gurney. I heard him call out to the ambulance driver. "Buddy, where's his ear?"

"What'd you mean?"

"Here." My father lifted away the bloodied mass of hair and torn tissue. "His whole ear has been ripped off."

"We just go scrape 'em off the road, Doc. It's up to you to patch 'em up, ain't it?"

"Not if I don't have all the parts. How about while I work on his wife, you get back out to the highway and see if you can scrape up an ear."

Buddy found the patient's missing ear, and my father painstakingly sutured it back on the man's head.

By the time I made it up to my father's office for the ride home, I was spent. Flopping down in a chair in his waiting room, I looked across at the only patient still there, an elderly lady who kept staring at me.

"You must be Dr. Mayo's boy," she said.

I nodded.

"You look so much like your father when he was your age." She fumbled with a package covered in newspaper resting against her knee. The woman had curly white hair with the curls spaced evenly around her head like the icing on a birthday cake.

"Thank you, ma'am." I buried my face behind a magazine.

"Your father saved my life. I had one of them ruptured appendixes. My neighbor told me if I'd waited another day longer, I wouldn't be here."

I lowered the magazine.

She peeled the newspaper off the package until I could see a painting. She lifted the painting and turned it in my direction. "It's the front of the hospital with your grandfather standing by his car," she said. "Do you think your father will like it?"

I squinted at the brightly colored painting, which was signed by Ina Bess Marchbanks in the lower right corner.

"Yes, ma'am," I said. How my father would respond to the painting, I had no idea.

She pushed herself up from her chair, the strain showing in her face, and slowly approached me.

"My husband and I have a place out by Reagor Springs where he raises cotton. He tries, bless his heart." Ina Bess straightened her homemade dress. Her eyes clouded. "This year he didn't do so good. So, I got nothing to pay your father with 'cept this." She held out the painting. "And I always pay my bills."

As we rode home in the car, the painting sat on the backseat. I tried to find out more about the purpose of the bulldozer behind the hospital, but like Ruby, my father claimed all he knew for sure were rumors. He'd heard nothing from the man himself, his own father.

When we got home, he lifted the painting gingerly out of the car and carried it securely in both hands. He nudged open the screen door with his foot, and by the look on his face, he couldn't have been more pleased. "Sweetheart," he called out to my mother. "Come see what Ina Bess Marchbanks painted for us."

"Who?" My mother asked.

"She lives out by Reagor Springs." He propped the painting on the kitchen counter and took a good hard look at it. "Her husband brings us the basket of corn each year."

"That's your payment for saving his arm?"

"It's all they have."

I said, "She said it was for taking out her appendix."

"You don't charge the doctors and their families," my mother said, eyeing my father. "You don't charge the nurses, the ministers. You don't charge the pharmacists."

"Or policemen," he said. "Or firemen, or dentists."

"And now you're adding farmers to the list?"

"Only in bad years," he said. "When they don't make a crop."

She stared at the painting leaning against the cabinet. "Would you mind telling me just who you do charge?"

"I don't know, exactly. You'll have to check with Dorothy."

Dorothy was my father's secretary, receptionist, and billing department rolled into one. He took care of the patients; she took care of all the rest. He had two unwritten rules he had gleaned from my grandfather: First, let patients pay what they can. Second, no collection agencies, no matter what.

He eased up behind my mother and put his arms around her. "Are we able to pay our bills?"

She nodded.

"Do we have a roof over our head and meals on the table?"

"We do."

He turned her around, "What more could we need?"

My mother didn't answer.

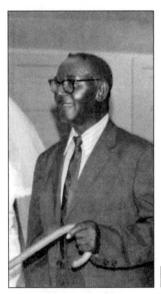

My father believed in getting to work early. The following day, we pulled into the hospital parking lot well before sunrise. I was a growing boy and required my sleep. My problem was that I needed a ride to work. With a flat tire on my bike and me too lazy to fix it, my father was the only driver going my way.

"See you this afternoon," he said, jumping out of the car for his early morning rounds.

I stayed behind and tried to catch a few minutes of sleep before my day began.

Gene Finley
Compliments of the Finley family

I awoke to see a man leaning against the hood of our car. I took a moment to recognize the face.

"Good morning, Robbie," Gene said. "These early morning hospital hours are hard on a growing boy." He turned his head to look at the bulldozer. The heavy machine had taken up residence behind the hospital about a week ago.

Gene was my grandfather's partner of sorts. He started at the hospital in the early 1920s, after the new building opened. He'd been there ever since. Although everyone agreed my grandfather ran the hospital in those early days, it was Gene who operated quietly behind the scenes to make things happen. I never saw them talk much, but Gene could sense when my grandfather needed something done. They were close, and so were our families, a rarity among the whites and Negroes at the time.

I slipped out of the car. "What's going on with the bulldozer?"

"Your grandfather has something you can't get from no school. Vision's what I call it. He knows what needs doing. Different from most folks around here, he does it. I've spent almost my whole life working with your grandfather." He nodded at the bulldozer. "When he's ready, he'll let us know what he's planning."

5

THE ROAD TO BOZ

———————— ∎ ————————

B y the time I changed into my scrubs and arrived at X-ray, Ruby
was already hard at work. Dr. Seichrest was due to arrive soon,
and Ruby planned to be ready.

"I asked Leon to have the first patient down here by seven-fifteen,"
she said. "We can shoot the plain films before the good doctor gets
here." She grabbed a cassette and loaded it into the bucky, a moveable
tray that slid under the table to hold the unexposed film.

"Do you want me to mix up the barium?" I asked.

"You know how Fancy Pants wants it, smooth with no lumps. Hell,
you'd think he was baking a cake. No, I'd wait until just before the
next patient has to drink it. A quick stir and down the hatch. I'm glad
it's not me."

"I'd rather take it that way than the other," I said, referring to the
barium enemas scattered throughout that morning.

Dr. Seichrest burst through the door. "It's that damned traffic," he
said. "Unpredictable. Either I'm too early or too late." He glanced at
Ruby, still adjusting the table. "Where's the first stiff?"

"You're thirty minutes early. Why don't you go grab a coffee?"

He caught sight of me. "You must be Mayo's boy. You favor him."

Dr. Leviticis Seichrest looked as if he'd stepped out of the Neiman

Marcus catalogue: three piece suit, matching tie and socks. No wrinkles. Two things set him apart from the men in the catalogue: his white-top shoes and his car. Dr. Seichrest drove a Bugatti, and he always parked at the far end of the parking lot. He claimed it was to avoid dents. I think he wanted to distance himself from the old clunkers in the lot.

"Yes, sir," I said.

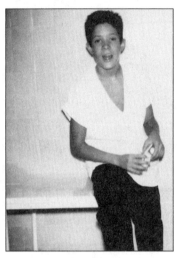

Rob Tenery
Photographer: Mayo Tenery, MD

"I always wondered why your father, with his Ivy-League training, chose to practice here."

"Maybe for the same reason you come down from Dallas."

He reached up and brushed lint from his lapel. "What do they call you?"

"Robbie," I said, but it didn't matter. Seichrest was gone.

Ruby said, "He's a good radiologist. Compared to the doctors who work in this hospital, I'm not sure 'good' is good enough."

Lucy Plummer was our third patient. She was also the wife of our postman. At fifty, she looked better than most women in Waxahachie. Unlike a lot of women in our small community who wore gloves and sipped tea, Lucy lived and worked on a small farm on the outskirts of town. On the day I last saw her at Trinity Pharmacy perched atop her stool at the soda fountain, every man in the place was staring in her direction. Today, as she lay on the stark examination table, a fluoroscopy screen overhead, she didn't look so pretty.

"Doctor," Lucy Plummer said, "that's enough, please. I can't take any more."

"Be still," Dr. Seichrest said. He loomed over her, poking on her exposed abdomen. "Be patient. We'll be through here in a few minutes." He reached over and unclamped the hemostat. Barium now flowed from the metal container down a long tube and into Lucy's rectum.

"I mean it. I can't take any more!" she shouted. "Please . . ."

"Another minute." Seichrest readjusted the fluoroscopy screen. He squinted and stared at the screen. "There." He clicked off the screen. "The rest is up to Mayo's boy, here."

And then, out Dr. Seichrest went, leaving Ruby and me alone with Mrs. Plummer.

Ruby flipped on the overhead lights.

My job was *evacuation*. Dr. Seichrest put the barium in; I let it out. As hospital duties went, it didn't get any lower than this. With three weeks of experience, I'd worked out a reasonably efficient evacuation system. My system was based on gravity. If I lowered the large metal canister below the X-ray table, the barium should flow out of the patient and back into the container. Then I would use a syringe to deflate the saline-filled balloon fixed to the end of the rubber tube that was secured deep inside the patient's rectum. If all went as planned, I'd be left with nothing but a few dribbles. The patient would expel any remaining barium liquid in the bathroom, and that was that.

I looked at Mrs. Plummer and then down at the metal canister on the floor beside the table. The canister should have been filled by now, yet it was empty.

"Could you push or something?" I asked, frustrated that my plan wasn't working.

"I'm trying," she groaned. "I need to go sooo . . . bad." She shifted on her side, but still nothing flowed back into the container. "Let me go in there." She pointed to the bathroom. "I know I can do it if I'm sitting up."

"But—" I said.

"Please," Mrs. Plummer said, her face contorted in pain.

"Okay, okay." I clamped the hemostat on the rubber tube and disconnected the tube from the container. "Now, ease off the table," I said. I held the tube above my head. "I'll follow you into the bathroom."

"What?"

"We don't have any other choice."

We were an odd pair, Mrs. Plummer clad in a hospital gown slit in the back with a rubber tube running out of her fanny, and I with the other end of the tube and a syringe in hand. We made it to the bathroom.

"Now sit down," I said, pointing my chin at the toilet. "I have to take the saline out of the balloon." My hands shook as I crammed the syringe into the small phalange that extended off the tube and drew back on the plunger.

Nothing came out!

"I can't hold it any longer," Mrs. Plummer yelled.

She lunged for the toilet. I felt a tug on the tube, a loud pop, and a stream of chalky yellow barium fluid shot out the back of Lucy Plummer's open gown. The mess coated the floors, walls, toilet, and everything else within a three-foot radius. Including me; I was drenched in the stuff.

Mrs. Plummer gave me a shove and slammed the door to the bathroom, leaving me to stand outside the door in a pool of excrement.

Just then, Dr. Seichrest sauntered in to the room, a cup of coffee in his hand. "Is the next patient ready yet?"

Fortunately, Willie took pity on me and drove me home to shower and change clothes. I took a long hot shower and washed away the entire mess. I wouldn't ever face Lucy Plummer again, front view or rear. By the time we arrived back at the hospital, Seichrest had left. I completed the rest of my shift in the solitude of the darkroom. Ruby brushed off the incident, claiming she had been in my position several times herself.

True or not, her words didn't make me feel any better.

At the end of the day, I ran into my grandfather.

He said, "Want to see how babies were delivered before we had hospitals? Hawkins and I have to run out to Boz. I have a patient out there about to have a baby, and she needs some help."

Dr. Hawkins was my grandfather's best friend. He was a general practitioner who had settled in Waxahachie just after the end of WWI.

"Let me check with my father," I said.

"Already have. Time's a-wastin'. We don't want her to have that baby without us."

The three of us sped along the chuckholed farm-to-market road. My grandfather and Dr. Hawkins talked to each other the way old men do, not so much to learn anything new as to confirm what they already knew.

"Old Bert must be close to seventy-five, wouldn't you say?" my grandfather said.

"Seventy-five sounds about right," Dr. Hawkins said.

"He's been raising crops and kids around here for as long as I can remember."

"I think Gerty is wife number three. Maybe we should ask what he's been drinkin' so we can get us some."

The endless rows of picked cotton fields whipped past our car. The smell of tilled earth and dried hay kept me comfortable in the backseat.

"Billy-Boy," Hawkins said, using my grandfather's nickname. "Riding out here on this dusty road reminds me of the time we picked up that cadaver in Dallas. You remember, we brought it back home to dissect."

"The time we picked up the farmer who ran out of gas?"

"That's the one."

"The poor soul climbed in the backseat and the body rolled on top of him. I'll bet he thought he'd met his maker."

"I can see it like it was yesterday," Hawkins said. "You took the corner too fast. The body fell over and the tarp slipped off."

"When he bailed from the car, I thought the poor fellow broke his neck. We were doing thirty-five, maybe more. He'd made it halfway across that cotton field before I could stop the car."

We topped a small rise. Dr. Hawkins yelled, "Billy, watch out!"

My grandfather slammed on the brakes. The tires screeched against the hot asphalt, I tumbled to the floor, and our car careened sideways before stopping ten feet from a large heifer lying stretched out in the road. The cow blocked our only access to a narrow one-lane bridge.

"What the hell?" my grandfather said.

I pulled myself back up onto the seat and watched as a wiry man clad in overalls approached our car. "Sorry about that. She's down with a calf." With a bloody hand, the man pointed at the cow. "She must have gotten spooked and jumped the fence."

"Move her," my grandfather said. "We've got to deliver a baby over at Bert's place."

"Not before she delivers, Doc. The calf is turned and way up in her and I ain't able to pull it out." The farmer showed us his bloody arm, as if to prove his point.

My grandfather grumbled under his breath and then pushed open the door and got out. Dr. Hawkins followed. I hung back by the car and watched while the two circled the cow.

"Billy-Boy, what do you think?" Hawkins asked, first looking at the cow, then glancing back at the car.

"I think we're at an impasse," he said. "There's no way around her." He pointed to the edge of the narrow bridge.

"You're not thinking about . . . ?" Dr. Hawkins said.

My grandfather nodded.

"Billy, you don't know anything about birthing a cow." He leaned back against the hood of our car, his foot propped up on the bumper.

"You and I have been delivering babies for years. How hard can it be? You just stick your hand up in there, grab anything you find, and pull it out."

"I keep hearing the word *you*, Billy-Boy."

My grandfather raised an eyebrow. He turned to the farmer kneeling next to his downed cow. "How tall are you?" he asked.

"Five-feet-six, maybe seven, without my boots."

"I'm five-feet-two," my grandfather said. He extended his arm to demonstrate it was shorter than the farmer's. He turned to Dr. Hawkins. "The other day you were bragging you were over six-feet. Now, why don't you hurry and roll up your sleeve. We have a baby to deliver."

With moral support from the three of us, Dr. Hawkins undertook the gory work of calf-birthing. Twenty minutes after the calf had safely emerged, we finally coaxed the heifer and her calf off the bridge and resumed our trip to Bert's farm near Boz.

My grandfather recommended that Dr. Hawkins hold his bloody arm out the window because of the blood and the stink. Even out the window, the set-up didn't sit well with me. No matter where I moved in the backseat, I was still downwind of the foul odor. As our car eased up the dirt road to Bert's farmhouse, I saw a man seated on the steps with a bundle in his lap.

The weathered structure, sorely in need of a new coat of paint, reminded me of Ollie's. The porch sat up off the ground and sagged in spots. The crawl space had several small animals tucked deep in the dark. The dank cubby hole was their hiding place to get out of the sun or for winter cold snaps, fall thunderstorms, and the occasional tornado.

"You're a little late, Doc," the man said. He lifted the newborn baby wrapped in a blanket. "Seems like there was no holdin' the little fella back when he made up his mind."

My grandfather and Dr. Hawkins, flushed with embarrassment, bolted out of the car.

"Where is she, Bert?" my grandfather asked. He snatched his medical bag out of the backseat.

"No need to hurry, Doc." He pushed himself to his feet carefully cradling the baby in his arms. "Mama came over and she's in there with Gerty, cleaning her up and getting rid of the afterbirth." Bert stepped aside as my grandfather disappeared into the house. Bert looked over at Dr. Hawkins' bloody arm. "What happened to you?"

"We had to stop off and do another delivery on the way," Dr. Hawkins said.

I half stumbled out of the car.

Bert said, "Does the boy there belong to you?"

"He's the Doc's grandson."

Bert turned to me. "You grow up to be a doctor like your granddad and you can take care of my boy someday. Mama made Gerty and me some beans and cornbread. Since you made the trip all the way out here to see us, it'd be downright unneighborly not to invite you inside for a bite." He waved me onto the porch. "Boy, I might even find a piece of pecan pie to go with that."

Dr. Hawkins stepped onto the porch.

Bert thrust out his free hand to stop him. "Nothing personal," his eyes darting to Hawkins' foul-smelling arm.

"I just need to wash up."

Bert pointed to the water-trough next to the barn. "Gerty's real particular about who comes in the house. How about I bring you a plate. You can eat out here."

Doctors, I was learning, sometimes get rewarded for their efforts in ways I never would have expected.

6

WHEN MEDICINE WAS A CALLING

W hile working at the hospital, I'd been able to set aside most of what I earned. In a few more weeks, I'd have enough to get the football I had been eyeing all summer. And with a new football, I reasoned, I'd somehow become more popular with the girls. My interest in girls had increased greatly in the last six months. Girls, however, hadn't shown the same interest in me. Without a girlfriend or a new football, I was left with ample time on my hands, time enough to begin to understand the peculiar rhythms of life at the hospital.

On Tuesday afternoon, an ambulance raced up to the hospital's emergency entrance. I poked my head out the door of X-ray as Buddy and his associate rushed a stretcher down the hall. Mrs. Delmer joined them, and all three disappeared through the swinging doors of the emergency room. I laid down my stack of films and followed.

Mrs. Delmer stood over a stretcher, her hands on her hips like a scolding schoolteacher.

"She told me it was an emergency," Buddy said.

"And the siren?" Mrs. Delmer asked.

"Look, we just haul 'em. It ain't up to me to make that decision."

"This is a hospital, not a dance hall. These people are sick or they wouldn't be here. They need their rest."

Everyone knew that Buddy was siren happy. He'd flip the switch at the slightest provocation. I'd heard rumors he even used the siren when he broke for lunch.

My father rushed into the room. "What do we have?"

"It's Ruth Stedware," Mrs. Delmer said, spinning toward my father. "Again!"

My father hunched over his patient. "Ruth," he said, his voice muted. "You can't keep doing this. We'll take care of you this time, but this is it." He straightened and signaled to Mrs. Delmer to carry on. He then said to Mrs. Stedware, "The ambulance is for real emergencies, not when you can't have a bowel movement."

Mrs. Stedware was the wife of a minister at the Baptist church. According to my father, there were several common problems with preachers' wives: They liked to ride in ambulances. They liked the special treatment. And they all had backaches, hemorrhoids, or they were constipated.

Mrs. Delmer nodded to Buddy. "Move her in there while I get the enema kit. Then you can take her back home. Without the siren." She glared at Buddy and his partner before disappearing into the supply room.

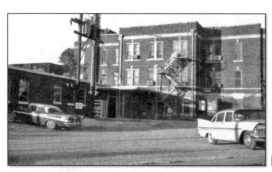

| The back parking lot at the hospital

By now, the bulldozer at the back of the hospital had finished clearing the shrubs and trees. The dozer was replaced with a half-dozen carpenters and laborers. In a few weeks, they had put up a one-story cinder-block building. On Friday, they had packed up and hauled off the last of their sawhorses and scaffolding. A cardboard sign affixed to the building's door read "Storage"–but I knew better. Each time I broached the subject with my father, he gave a vague answer that the hospital needed room to expand. He said the board of directors hadn't made a final determination how to use the extra space.

At the end of the day, I eased across the dusty parking lot and over to the new building. The door was closed, but I turned the knob and it clicked open. "Is anyone here?"

When I got no reply, I slipped inside. The building was divided into two areas. I made my way into a large room filled with boxes and furniture stacked against the wall. Most of it was disassembled bed frames and mattresses. A dozen or so wooden vegetable crates sat in the far corner, identical to those I'd seen in the back room at the Cotton Club.

Then I saw it. A freshly painted sign over the door read "Men's Ward."

Behind me, a man said, "Who is that in here?"

"It's me," I answered, barely able to coax out a response.

Gene stood there. His angry stare melted when he recognized me. "What are you doing? Don't you know you're not supposed to be in here?"

"I wasn't sure. I was just . . ."

"Well, you're not. Not until your grandfather says everything's okay."

"I don't understand."

"I can't expect you to," he said. "My people have waited a long time for this day." His voice trailed off as he moved back into the other room labeled "Women's Ward."

"When does it open?"

"Soon, I hope. Soon."

Shortly thereafter, I stopped by my father's office, but he wasn't in. I slipped through the waiting room across the hall and tapped on the door to my grandfather's office. I heard a muffled reply and pushed open the door.

"What is it?" my grandfather said.

"I wanted to thank you for taking me out to Bert and Gerty's."

Then I saw my father leaning against the wall.

My grandfather grunted. He turned back toward my father and said, "I've never had to do one before." He waved a cigar butt in his fingers like a baton. "It's an embarrassment."

"The baby is too big for a D&C," my father said. "It's been dead for over a week and she hasn't aborted the fetus on her own. I'll have to do a C-section. That or give him a call."

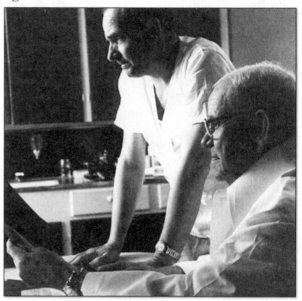

Dr. Mayo and Dr. W. C.
Compliments of the Amon Carter Museum
Photographer: Nell Dorr

"It'll cause scarring. If she gets pregnant again, she'll need another C-section. She's only twenty." My grandfather frowned at the patient's chart. "Aborting is the only answer." He picked up the phone, flipped open the telephone book, and ran his finger down the page until he reached Paxton, C. L. MD He called out the number to the operator. "After all I've done to try to put him out of business, now I'm asking for help. All because I haven't been trained to do an abort . . ."

Dr. C. L. Paxton was a salty old general practitioner who had been doing illegal abortions ever since coming to Ellis County more than thirty years ago. He was proficient at the task, and except for a six-month stint at the state prison in Huntsville, he had been able to avoid prosecution despite repeated complaints against him. The old doctor held an odd place in our community. Publicly, he was disdained by the town's citizens. However, when their daughters needed help, they'd come to Dr. Paxton in the dead of night. For my grandfather to ask for assistance from Paxton was against the Hippocratic Oath, as he saw it. It was also a devastating blow to his pride.

"Clarence. W. C. here," my grandfather said into the phone. "Mayo and I have a patient with some difficulty. We were wondering if we might get your advice." He was selecting his words carefully. "I know it's been a long time since we last spoke." My grandfather reached up and tugged at his shirt collar. "Unfortunately, we do have our differences."

Dr. Paxton spoke into the phone.

"A large Foley catheter," my grandfather repeated. "Two-hundred and fifty cc's of normal saline." He reached for his cigar. "Thanks for the advice, Clarence."

Paxton said something and the phone went dead.

My grandfather placed the phone back in its cradle.

"What'd he say?" my father asked.

"He said, he hoped I'd remember we're both physicians."

"That's it?"

"And I needed to understand something: just because the legal system hadn't caught up to his line of thinking, he was still trying to help his patients."

My father never mentioned whether he acted on Dr. Paxton's advice. His silence on the subject told me all he wanted me to know: his patient's health came first.

* * *

My grandfather did not approve of old Dr. Paxton, but he was also distressed by young doctors "without passion."

Dr. Barry Mendelson was a good example and one of Ellis County's most colorful physicians. Born into poverty, he had excelled in school while holding down a full-time job at the local hardware store. My grandfather, always sympathetic to the underdog—probably because of his own humble beginnings as a pharmacy apprentice in Pulaski, Tennessee—took Mendelson under his wing. He had recommended Mendelson for medical school and even helped him get a scholarship to pay the tuition. When the young physician returned to Ellis County to set up practice, everyone expected him to keep with his habit of hard work and humility. It didn't happen.

According to my grandfather, Mendelson had become one of a new

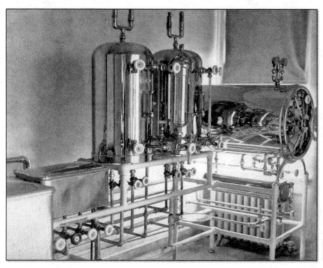

*Autoclaves at
the hospital*

generation of doctors without passion. Desire to make some money, yes; ambition, even; but very little passion for medicine or patients. "The more medical schools focused on science," he told me, "the less attention they paid to the art of healing."

Mendelson's first purchase as a physician was a two-hundred dollar, custom-made, silk suit tailored in Dallas. To go with it, he bought two Bronzini ties. After his first six months in practice, he put a down payment on a brand-new, dark-brown Lincoln Continental with more chrome than the autoclaves in surgery. He parked the car out front of his office for all to see. That was when he wasn't at the Country Club boasting how busy he was back at the office.

Mendelson often referred patients to the hospital for X-rays, which is how I first met him.

Ruby Profit took a call and told me they needed one of us over in the emergency room. When Ruby said "one of us," she usually meant me.

"What can I do to help?" I asked.

"They need the portable machine."

I hurried across the room and tugged the old X-ray machine from its place in the corner.

"Mendelson referred a patient over with shortness of breath and fever," she said. "Take a chest X-ray. The note from Mendelson's nurse said to run the films by your father."

I struggled to get the bulky machine into the emergency room. "Where's the patient?"

The nurse pointed at a pale, thin woman wrapped in a blanket lying on the exam table. The woman thrust the note from Mendelson's office at me. "He said Dr. Mayo would take a look at me. Dr. Mendelson said he was always here."

I carefully slid the unexposed X-ray cassette under her back.

"If Dr. Mayo has any questions," she said, "Dr. Mendelson said the operator in Ennis knew how to get in touch with him."

I had a lot to learn, but even then I understood that for some doctors, medicine was a means to a better life and nothing more. For these doctors, medicine was a job, a nine-to-five whose primary rewards were prestige and money. The doctors I had grown to respect without knowing it, like my grandfather and father and others, recognized that the profession of medicine was much more. For these men, medicine was an inner impulse and a conviction of divine influence. Medicine was their calling.

7

Medical Miracles

—————— ▪ ——————

I took the stairs up to my father's office.

"He's just finished the last patient," Dorothy said.

I opened the door to his inner office. The acrid smell of cigarette smoke swept around me. "Come in," he said. He muffled a cough into his closed fist. "Shut the door behind you."

"Is this about the trip?" One of my father's former patients had given us the use of his beach house in Galveston for a week. I couldn't wait.

"I hear you had a visit with Gene?"

"Well, yes . . . I was curious is all."

He coughed again. "You weren't supposed to be there. But since you've been inside, you know the building was never intended for storage." He eased back in his chair. "The board of directors has decided that Gene's people deserve better than the back room at the Cotton Club."

"The board of directors?" I recalled the rumor that my grandfather had given them an ultimatum.

"Let's just say they were able to see the light."

"Why not add a wing on to the hospital?" I asked.

"The community isn't ready for that."

Someone knocked on the office door. "Yes?" my father said.

"Dr. Mayo!" Dorothy pushed through the door. "They need you in the emergency room. Now!"

"What is it?"

"A young girl has been run over by a motorboat. She's hurt bad."

In the emergency room, I shivered at the gruesome sight. If my father hadn't needed all available hands to pump blood, I would have retreated to X-ray. The girl, barely in her teens, lay on the examination table with blood streaming out of giant lacerations on her back and buttocks.

"More packing!" my father called out to the two nurses. The nurses struggled to control the young girl's bleeding. "Here, Robbie," he said. "Come up and hold these while I get the IVs started."

I pressed the sterile gauze pads into the girl's deep wounds, trying to staunch her loss of blood.

The girl was Ashley Hargrove, the younger sister of a boy in my Cub Scout troop. She looked up at me.

"Please help me," she whispered. Her voice trailed off as she lapsed into semi-consciousness.

I pressed harder, knowing it was all the help I could offer. That and reassurance. "You're going to be all right."

My father nudged me aside. "Go help pump blood." He nodded to the far end of the table where two IV stands had been set up. "I'll take over here."

At that moment I understood that the man standing beside me was not only my father, but a physician whose hands were guided by a spiritual force greater than his own.

When we arrived home, the meal my mother had stored in the refrigerator no longer concerned me. After ten pints of blood and more sutures than I could count, Ashley had made it through surgery. Her blood pressure was low, and that worried my father. He discussed with my grandfather the possibility of evacuating her to Dallas and even put in a call to a specialist at Baylor Hospital. The two of them agreed the ambulance ride could kill her. After a few quick bites of my mother's leftover supper, my father returned to the hospital.

Close to midnight, the phone rang. My mother answered. I lay in bed and listened to her muffled voice. My suitcase was on the floor beside my bed, packed for our Galveston trip. She said, "I'll tell them," disappointment evident in her voice. "Want me to bring you out a clean set of clothes?"

I got out of bed and poked my head into her bedroom. "What did he say?"

"Ashley is no better."

"Is that what you were supposed to tell us?" I asked and moved into the bedroom so I wouldn't wake up my sister asleep down the hall.

"We're not going." Her voice was barely a whisper.

"Where?"

"To Galveston. She's too sick, and your father feels he can't leave her."

"But that's our family vacation! Can't someone else take over for him?"

"Probably," she said. Then she sat up on the edge of the bed. "When your father and I got married, he asked me not to make him choose between me and his patients."

"So his patients are more important than his family?"

"No. I think it means if that young girl has anything going for her, it's that your father is her doctor."

Ashley died that night.

My mother didn't wake me with the news. At the breakfast table, I found my father, still in scrubs, slumped over his coffee. After he told me, I felt overwhelmed and went back to bed. The loss took a whole day out of me. That evening, my father led me into the living room and sat me down on the couch beside him. "I'm sorry about Galveston. It's all right to feel bad about Ashley, but as long as you know you did your best, you just have to go on. We'll leave for the hospital at six in the morning. Same as usual."

I didn't answer, but I don't think he expected one.

The next morning, when we pulled into the hospital parking lot, I saw Gene leaning into the open trunk of his car.

"Flat tire?" I called out.

"Nope."

I moved closer and peeked over his shoulder. His trunk was loaded with baskets full of fresh vegetables. I eased around beside him when he lifted one for me to see.

"I grew them myself," he said. "Even nursed them through the hot summer, so they wouldn't burn up."

"What are you planning to do with them?"

"Got a free pair of hands?"

I grabbed one of the baskets, inhaling the smell of freshly gathered sweet potatoes. By the time I looked up, Gene had started toward the back door to the new building.

"Everybody gives in different ways," he said. "Your grandfather . . . well, if it wasn't for him, that building wouldn't be here." Gene laid his basket down. "Got a minute?"

I nodded.

Gene headed for the new building and I followed, my arms still wrapped around the heavy basket. When we reached the door, Gene unlocked it and we pushed on in.

"Leave them there," he said, signaling for me to put down the basket. He flipped on the lights and smiled. "Take a real look around, why don't you."

The transformation shocked me. The litter, dust, and scattered debris from days before had been swept clean. In each ward, fresh sheets and pillows finished out the beds. Two large fans affixed to the ceilings, each with its own set of lights, brought the freshly painted room to life. "I can't believe it," I said. I noticed the stands that acted as partitions between the beds. They had fresh white linen cloths covering the tops, just like at the Cotton Club. But what lay before me were now white-enameled metal stands identical to the ones in the main hospital. "What happened to the crates?"

Gene moved over to the rear door and pushed it open. "Take a look-see." He pointed to stacks of stained wooden vegetable boxes—the same containers I'd seen piled to the ceiling in the men's ward days before—sitting in the trash area.

"The bedside tables we got inside, they came yesterday. They were a gift from the people in my church." He pulled the door closed. "Robbie, we don't have much, but my people gives what they can." His eyes drifted over to the basket of freshly picked vegetables I had set by the front door. "Now, before you go to work, why don't you help me get those vegetables over to the kitchen?"

Miracles come in many forms. To Gene, the new building was just such a miracle. To patients like Livia Moore, a miracle meant briefly stepping over that fine line between life and death.

Already prepped for her routine appendectomy, Mrs. Moore passed the first test: she didn't wince when the pointed towel clips pierced her skin to hold the sterile drapes in position. The iodine prep released a potent medicinal smell throughout the operating room.

I pulled a stool to the foot of the table.

The circulating nurse and her assistant spoke quietly. My father hummed. His humming was a sign that all was well. He held out his hand as the circulating nurse slapped the scalpel into his palm. With the steel blade poised just inches above Mrs. Moore's exposed abdomen, he gave one final glance at Oma Jones.

"Ready?" he asked.

Oma was silent. She was buried behind a sterile drape affixed with hemostats to two IV poles.

"Are we ready to start the procedure, Oma?" he asked again.

"I'm not getting a pulse, Dr. Mayo."

My father moved to the head of the table. "What's her blood pressure?"

"Sixty over forty, and that was about a minute ago."

"Turn off the anesthetic!" My father grabbed Oma Jones' stethoscope, then probed Livia Moore's chest for any sign of a heartbeat. "Get these drapes off."

Livia Moore's lips were blue, her pallor stark. My father raised his closed fist and pounded on Livia Moore's exposed chest. The team surrounding my father waited as he checked again for a pulse. He shook his head and began rhythmically pushing on her chest. Oma Jones forced oxygen into the patient's lungs through the endotracheal tube.

"Draw up the intracardiac epinephrine." He looked at the circulating nurse. "Get out the chest set, just in case."

I hopped off my stool and pulled it away from the operating table.

The nurse handed my father a small syringe with the long needle. He carefully placed his fingers on Livia Moore's chest and thrust the needle into her skin all the way to the hub. The syringe empty, he extracted the needle and handed it to the scrub nurse. Again, he checked for a pulse. Nothing! My father grabbed a gauze sponge, dipped it in the bowl of iodine prep, and wiped it across Livia Moore's bare chest. He picked up the scalpel and plunged it deep into her chest, opening up an eight-inch incision. Only a small amount of dark blood oozed from the wound. His gloved hand disappeared inside her chest. For five long minutes, he squeezed her heart, until the pinkish color returned to Livia Moore's body.

As life returned to Mrs. Moore, I felt that in a some small way, I'd contributed to her recovery by just being there. And I'd come to appreciate the importance of the medical team.

Slowly, my father pulled his hand from her chest as her separated ribs closed behind him. He looked up at Oma Jones.

"Blood pressure ninety-five and rising. Her pulse is hovering around eighty." A smile peeked out through the edges of her surgical mask.

My father glanced at the circulating nurse. "Get me a fresh gown and a new set of gloves. We still have her chest to close and an appendix to remove before we call it a day."

The operation was a success. Now for the hard part.

He hesitated outside the door to Mrs. Moore's hospital room. "I wanted to wait until she was fully awake," my father said.

"I don't understand," I said.

"To explain it to her. To explain what happened in surgery. The family took it pretty well, being that she's alive." He grinned weakly and then glanced back at the door. "She's going to ask why her heart stopped, and I'm going to give her the same answer I've given since I walked on the wards as an intern—there's still so much in medicine we have yet to understand."

My father looked edgy, his face drawn. Normally, I didn't accompany him on morning rounds, but I wanted to see how Mrs. Moore would take the news. I hung back by the door, as he quietly moved into her darkened room.

"Livia," he said "How are you feeling this morning?"

"Oh Dr. Mayo," she said, her voice thready. "I'm so sore."

"That's to be expected. Your surgery was just yesterday." He gently pulled back the bedcovers and raised her hospital gown, exposing the two bandages wrapped across her body. She had a small bandage across her lower abdomen and a much larger one across her chest. "You know what they say. It always hurts more the second day."

I could see his fingers working at the edge of the smaller bandage, slowly freeing it from her skin.

"There," he said. He lifted the bandage and dropped it in the wastebasket beside her bed. "I'll have Mrs. Delmer come in and dress those again. This time the bandages will be smaller."

Mrs. Moore shivered. She reached for the sheet that was pushed down below her navel.

"You'll notice that you have two incisions. One where I took out your appendix, and another." My father cleared his throat. "You had a cardiac arrest during surgery yesterday."

Mrs. Moore didn't look at him. She stared off to a darkened corner of the room. Her mind must have been in another place where bad things didn't happen to good people. I could read it in her face, a resignation and acceptance. She stayed that way for a long time. She took a deep breath and said, "You mean my heart stopped?"

"Exactly. That's the reason for the large incision on your chest. It looks ugly now, but in time the scar will fade. Besides, only your husband will see it anyway." He forced a smile.

A long, uncomfortable pause passed between them. "You saved my life?"

"I guess I did."

She gazed up at him. "Well, what do you know?"

8

GIVING MOTHER NATURE A CHANCE

S till short of cash with the start of high school less than a week
away, I extended my job at the hospital. I'd come to appreciate
the dedication it took to become a doctor. My father and
grandfather set the bar high when it came to professional standards,
and I had serious doubts I could live up to those standards.

I wasn't the only one.

A new physician moved to the area, and rather than rely on old-
school word-of-mouth to build his practice, he took out a flashy
advertisement in the *Daily Light*, Waxahachie's local newspaper.

My father and grandfather hunched over the desk and glared at the
newspaper. The two of them squinted at a four-by-five inch box in the
lower corner of the paper.

"If he gets away with it," my father said. "It'll only be a matter of time.
He and those like him will turn this profession into a bunch of high-paid
technicians. His kind are willing to sell their souls for a few extra bucks."

"Never heard of him," my grandfather said.

"He just opened his office." My father sat in the chair at the side of
the desk.

I moved forward to get a better look. The advertisement said that
Charles P. Sturgess, MD, a world-renowned surgeon and lecturer, had

opened a new practice in Waxahachie. He promised to use the latest technology, and he was offering a 50 percent discount to the first twenty-five patients to call for an appointment. There was more, but that was the gist of it.

My father pulled out a wrinkled paper from his pocket. "I called Bob Heaton, the executive director at the Dallas County Medical Society, to see if he could turn up any information on Sturgess." Unfolding the sheet, he laid it on the desk.

The standard newspaper announcement for a new doctor was a tasteful one-by-two inch box with the name, area of interest, office hours, and address. That's it, nothing more. Sturgess had broken with tradition. Worse, he offered a discount.

"Heaton was able to track him down through the State Board of Medical Examiners," my father said. "He's recently off probation for over-prescribing narcotics."

"Where's he from?" my grandfather asked.

"His last office was Houston. They kicked him out for ethics violations. According to Heaton, Sturgess gave a lecture in Brazil, but it had to do with a rare tropical disease he'd seen as a resident." My father continued, "Most of those who attended probably didn't speak English. As for the rest of the world, I was told he's never been much east of the Mississippi."

My grandfather laid down the newspaper and put his half-chewed stogie back in his mouth. "Where does he plan to do his surgery?"

"Here at the hospital. His attorney came by to pick up an application yesterday."

"His attorney! What did you tell him?"

"It's a her. She's out of some high-priced law firm in Dallas. I explained that Dr. Sturgess first had to be accepted as a member of our county medical society before he could join the hospital staff. She claimed medical societies were just good-old-boy organizations, and being a member had nothing to do with her client's ability to practice medicine."

My grandfather spit a bit of tobacco at his wastebasket. "You did tell her those were the rules before I arrived? And that they were set down to protect patients."

"She said we were behind the times. If I didn't understand, she'd be glad to explain it to me in court."

"Makes you wonder what we're coming to, if we let a doctor like this loose on our patients."

━━━ ■ ━━━

My father had a natural instinct for scoundrels like Dr. Sturgess. He also knew that he didn't have all the answers. When a problem was outside his area of expertise, he wasn't above asking for help. When Veda Sneed was admitted to the hospital with intermittent bowel obstruction, that's just what he did.

Veda Sneed was still up to her old ways, demanding that Willie transport her to and from her appointments throughout the hospital. Miss Sneed had finally agreed to let my father do the surgery if my grandfather supervised—if an operation was absolutely necessary. My father took it as a sign he had come of age, as far as the old Waxahachie was concerned. Ruby and I took X-rays of Miss Sneed's upper and lower intestinal system, yet no one could locate a blockage.

My father peered over Dr. Seichrest's shoulder as the radiologist reviewed her films.

"Mayo, I don't know what else to tell you," Seichrest said, his finger tracing the intricate crevices of Sneed's small bowel. "She must have a stricture in there somewhere, but I'll be damned if it shows up on these X-rays. You may just have to go in there and take a look around."

"That would make this her third operation, which just sets her up for more adhesions. I've had the Miller-Abbot tube in her since she's been here and every time I clamp it off, she bloats right back up." My father said, "I debated calling Marion Fuquay to see if he would come down and have a look at her."

"Fuquay, the father of GI surgery?" Seichrest asked, his tone unbelieving. "What makes you think he'd come all the way from Philadelphia to Waxahachie to see one of your patients?"

"I'm one of his boys," my father said. "I did two years of my residency under him. He's in Dallas for a seminar at the medical school."

Seichrest turned up one corner of his mouth, as if he weren't buying it. That was all it took. My father was on the phone with Dr. Fuquay within minutes and the two had arranged that Dr. Fuquay would drive down and take a look at Miss Sneed.

—————

On our way back to the hospital that evening after dinner, my father was more than jovial. He was euphoric that his mentor was coming to visit.

"This guy is the expert," my father said. We pulled into the hospital's darkened parking lot. I could tell by his fingers drumming on the steering wheel, he was nervous. Like his peers, my father wanted to prove he could offer anything the Dallas doctors could. "Just hang back and don't get in the way," he said.

Dr. Fuquay was already waiting, sitting in a wheelchair by the emergency room entrance. "Finished early," he said, hopping up. He was nearly bald, a bespectacled man in a crumpled brown suit and scuffed wingback shoes. His authoritative voice was confident and clear. "I once thought about locating here in Texas," he said, "but when we came down to look around, my wife wouldn't have it. Her family goes back five generations in and around Boston. I guess she couldn't get that far away from her roots. Mayo, your wife was from up East somewhere?"

"Florida and Connecticut," my father said. "It took some adjustment on her part, but it's worked out well."

"I guess she was a little more adventuresome than my wife." Fuquay looked over at me. "Is that your boy?"

I nodded.

He grinned at me. "Let's go have a look at your father's patient."

After a quick review of Miss Sneed's X-rays, we made it to her room. My father drawled on about the tests he had run and the number of times he had clamped and unclamped the Miller-Abbot tube that ran from the patient's nose to her stomach.

Fuquay listened attentively. "What are you hungry for, Miss Sneed?"

"I don't know what you mean."

"If you could have anything you wanted to eat right now, what would it be?"

"Strawberry ice cream," she said, her lips parched and scaly. I didn't know if it was because of her illness or malnourishment from having the tube in her stomach for the last several days, but it was obvious Miss Sneed had lost much of the imperiousness that kept us all jumping.

"Mayo, do you think you can get Miss Sneed some strawberry ice cream?"

"Yes. I suppose we could, but—"

"Let's give it a try." Dr. Fuquay reached for the wastebasket beside the bed and pulled it up close. "Now Miss Sneed, let's get this thing out." He gently pulled on the long, rubber tube as it slid out of her stomach and back up her esophagus. The red hose was covered in slimy, green mucous. "Isn't that better?" he asked, dropping the putrid tube into the wastebasket.

"Why?" was all my father could manage.

"Well, Mayo, Miss Sneed's body knows what it needs. Let's let her eat, encourage her to be normal. What's the worst that can happen, we put the tube back in and have to open her up?"

As it turns out, Dr. Fuquay's treatment paid off.

With the strawberry ice cream, Miss Sneed's obstructed bowel slowly opened. My father's diagnosis had been correct; however, he hadn't relied enough on Mother Nature to work out the kinks in the human alimentary system. The experience taught me a useful lesson: doctors never stop being students.

───── ▬ ■ ▬ ─────

August in Texas is typically dry, but that August a rogue cool front swept down from western Canada, collided with the moist air coming out of the Gulf, and produced a trough of thunderstorms like I'd never seen. As I hiked to the surgery suite, I could see torrents of rain through the windows and an ominous dark green tint to the sky. In the hall, I saw Willie positioning his empty gurney against the wall.

"Pretty bad out there," I said. "Maybe tornado weather."

"It don't matter to me. We is like the Postal Service around here. Nothing stops us. Not rain, nor snow, nor . . . I forget how the rest of it goes."

I changed into a fresh set of scrubs, grabbed a mask, and tied it on. I moved into the operating room where my father and grandfather had begun surgery on Hanna McCartney's broken hip.

"Put her films up on the view-box," my father said. He stood at the operating table, his voice truncated by a blast of thunder. The lights flickered.

"That was close," I said.

My grandfather held a bloody sponge over the open wound on the side of Hanna McCartney's hip. "I've played golf in worse weather." He raised his bloodied hand above his head making it the highest point in the room. He was challenging the thunderstorm to strike him. His indifference to adversity was typical Dr. W. C. A thunderstorm was nothing to a man who journeyed from Tennessee to Texas in a covered wagon, all before he was twenty-five.

I put up the X-rays and stood back out of the way.

For the next thirty minutes, my grandfather pulled on retractors while my father cut, sawed, and pounded on

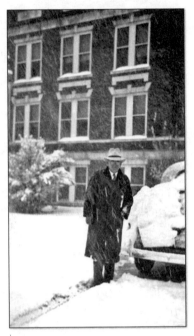

Dr. W. C.

bone to remove the head of Mrs. McCartney's broken femur. They replaced it with an artificial one. Undaunted by the rain against the windows, my grandfather bantered with the OR staff.

"Yesterday was the last time I throw a club in the lake," he said.

"Is that so," my father said.

"Too expensive. Besides, I go out there to relax. I have to remember golf is a game."

"So what about throwing instruments?"

My grandfather chuckled. "On that I make no commitments."

An explosion of light poured through the window. A moment later thunder pounded the walls and knocked the empty jacket of X-rays out of my hands. The operating room went dark. Except for the tapping of rain on the windows, we stood paralyzed in silence.

"What the hell?" my grandfather said.

"I guess you won't be testing your resolution at the Country Club today." My father's quip died in the darkness as we waited for the lights to come back on. "Oma?" His tone turned serious. "How are you doing up there?"

"Okay for now," she said. She had a small flashlight in her hand. "But we're in trouble if the lights don't come back on soon."

Anesthesia was tricky. Turn off the gas and Hanna McCartney wakes up in the middle of surgery; leave her under for too long and who knows what might happen. For an elderly patient like Mrs. McCartney, whose physical state was fragile at best, too much anesthesia could kill her.

"Get that flashlight up here," my father said. "What about the emergency pack?"

"We sent them out last week for repairs. The loaner they promised hasn't arrived."

My father looked at the patient's open wound. "I can't see enough to finish up."

"Looks like you may have no other choice," my grandfather said.

"Dr. Mayo," the nurse said. "I'll go see what I can do."

She turned to leave, when the operating room doors swung open.

Gene stood in the darkness, his rain-drenched clothes dripping puddles on the floor. "I thought you might be needing this."

Gene, puffing hard, struggled to push an IV pole with two giant light bulbs strapped to the top with tape. He held a heavy square box under his other arm.

"Where'd you get that?" my grandfather asked.

"I made it." He leaned over and set the box on the floor with a thud. "Out of some things I found here at the hospital. And my car battery."

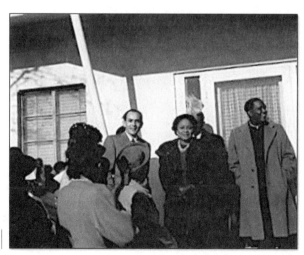

Dr. Mayo at the opening
of the Annex

The lights worked fine. My father finished twisting in the last screw in Mrs. McCartney's new hip and sutured the incision. He put the final touches to her bandage then turned around to Gene. "Thanks for what you did."

Gene flushed at my father's praise. "No need for that, Doc. I do need one thing, though."

The screwdriver still in his hand, my father hesitated. "What is it?"

Gene looked down at the car battery on the floor. "A ride home."

Hanna McCartney was the first patient admitted to the Annex—the Negroes-only addition out back. Establishing the Annex was an accomplishment my grandfather was fiercely proud of, though you couldn't tell it by him. He kept much of his thoughts to himself. Even when he did get his way, as he usually did, he didn't rub it in people's noses. The Annex was a win for my grandfather, but it was a bigger win for the black folks of Waxahachie. After a lifetime of dedication to her people, Priscilla retired her nurse's uniform when the last patient was discharged from the Cotton Club and admitted to the Annex.

9

ALL PATIENTS UNDER ONE ROOF

High school was a whole new experience. Although the teachers expected more of me, the girls in my class and the upper classmen treated me like I was still in the eighth grade. Most of my buddies experienced the same thing. A handful of friends and I formed a fraternity of losers and spent a great deal of time playing backyard football. My social life improved once I got my driver's license, which enabled me to get to our football games and, theoretically, to go on a date. The problem with dating was that high school girls wanted to go out with juniors and seniors, which I was not. And most of the eighth-grade girls couldn't date without a chaperone, a condition that sapped my enthusiasm.

At Christmas break, I reluctantly agreed to devote one of my free weeks to working in X-ray while Ruby took a long-overdue vacation to visit her family in Ohio. Since I wasn't certified, all elective procedures were cancelled in her absence. But because the sick and injured never took a holiday, there was still plenty to do.

On my first morning working alone, my father poked his head through the door to X-ray.

"Think you could spare me a couple of hours this afternoon? Minnie Bounds is back in with a hernia. I could use an extra pair of hands.

Who knows? Someday I might be holding retractors for you."

I was a one-man-show for the week, so I had to think before answering.

"I should have all the filing done by then," I said.

Minnie Bounds was a large woman. Some time ago, Miss Bounds stepped on the scales over at the cotton gin. She came in close to six-hundred and fifty pounds. She claimed her size was a glandular problem. My father said her only problem was her elbow—it kept allowing her hand to her mouth. I was eager to see how she was going to fit on the operating table, since it stood only eighteen inches wide.

Rushing through my chores, I made it over to surgery in time to scrub up. I could see Miss Bounds straddling two operating tables that had been roped together at the bottom. At the head of the table, Oma Jones prepared to put Miss Bounds to sleep.

Miss Bounds noticed me. "Is your boy going to help you today?"

"I brought him in for reinforcements."

"Dr. Mayo, while you're in there, why don't you take out the tapeworm in my stomach, so I don't feel so hungry all the time?"

Oma Jones clamped the mask over her face. "Now count backwards from a hundred and the next thing you know, you'll be in the recovery room waking up."

Although I had helped my father in surgery before, it was only with minor procedures, setting fractures, and examining lumps and bumps. I basically washed my hands and threw on some gloves. Today, I went through the required five-minute prep—three hundred seconds of hell as the bristles of the scrub brush scraped into the skin of my hands and forearms. My father had lectured me on the importance of sterility, but I was convinced his lengthy scrub policy was a test to see if I was cut out to be a surgeon.

"Towel," I called out. A scrub nurse scurried over and handed me a towel.

I stepped up on the footstool. Minnie's giant abdomen was a daunting sight with its endless rolls of fat. I wondered how far down my father would have to dig to find the hernia.

He held up the scalpel and looked over at me. "Ready?"

I nodded, proud that he finally trusted me enough to stand across the table from him.

He pressed the sharp blade deep into her flesh and extended the wound down past her navel. Mounds of yellow fat burst forward. The fat was dotted with ripples of bright red blood. He pressed a large gauze pad into the open wound and thrust out his hand.

"Hemostat."

I was determined to show Oma Jones I could stand the sight of blood and that my father's trust was justified. My job was to hold back Minnie's fat. An unglamorous task; nonetheless, I felt part of the team.

"What do you want me to do?" I asked.

My father looked over at me. "If my feet start to disappear, just grab hold of me."

It was a smirky joke, but I think even Minnie might have given up a chuckle.

After surgery, I rushed back to X-ray. Just as I returned, I got a call from a nurse.

"Miss Thorne refuses to come down there. She said the hospital is full of sick people. They've got germs and she doesn't want to leave her room. She told me to tell you, 'If you want an X-ray, you'll have to do it up here'."

Edna Thorne had been my third-grade teacher. Even in those days, she was considered eccentric, bringing all her food and water from home rather than eating with the rest of us. I could imagine the shock this hospitalization was having on her system.

"Tell her I'll bring the portable machine."

By the time I made it to her room, it was after three o'clock.

"Is that you, Robbie?" Miss Thorne asked.

I struggled to maneuver the large machine through her door. "Yes, ma'am."

Miss Thorne spoke in her teacher's voice. "I hope you're qualified to operate that machine."

"Yes, ma'am."

"Please tell me you washed your hands before you got here. With the Annex over here, you can't be too careful."

"Yes, ma'am."

"What are you now, fifteen?"

"Close," I said. "Can I get you to hold this against your chest and turn around with your feet hanging off the edge of the bed?" I reached out with the heavy film cassette.

She recoiled. "Have you scrubbed that down with alcohol? For all I know, it was used over in the Annex." She pointed to a large bottle of alcohol resting on her bedside stand. "I brought it from home, just in case."

Moving over to the small table, I removed one of her tissues and dabbed it with the alcohol. "What are you in for?"

"Your grandfather is supposed to remove my gallbladder." She relaxed as she watched me clean the X-ray cassette. "When I got here, he found I was anemic. Said he could give me iron to build me up, but if I waited too long, there would be a good chance I would have another attack. So he's going to give me a transfusion first."

I tossed the tissue in the wastebasket and handed her the cassette. "There, clean as a whistle."

"What about your hands?"

Enough was enough. I ignored Miss Thorne's question and repositioned the X-ray cassette. "Who in your family is going to donate the blood?"

She held the unexposed film tightly against her chest. "They're all gone. I do have a cousin near San Antonio, but we haven't spoken in years. Your grandfather said the laboratory keeps a list of donors for situations like mine. I think they've already called someone. They'll be in this afternoon, since my surgery is scheduled for in the morning." She hunched over the large cassette. "Hurry up. This thing is uncomfortable. Now, I didn't hear your answer about washing your hands before you came up here."

"I just . . ."

I heard feet shuffling behind me. I noticed a colored man, dressed in his Sunday suit. The jacket was too small and the pants too short, but the outfit was clean and recently pressed. He paused at the door, coughed to get our attention, and spoke in a low whisper, like people unfamiliar with hospitals often do. "Would you please tell me where y'alls laboratory is at?" The man stood uncomfortably in the doorway to Miss Thorne's room, unsure exactly what to do with his hands. "They tell me someone needs my blood."

72

I pointed down the hall.

"Thank you, kindly."

It took thirty minutes to lug the bulky machine back down to X-ray, develop the film, and bring the wet film up to my grandfather. I slid Miss Thorne's chest X-ray onto the view-box in his office.

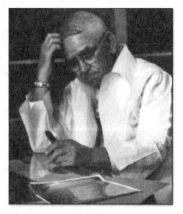

Dr. W. C.
Compliments of the Amon Carter Museum
Photographer: Nell Dorr

"I had to shoot it with the portable," I said. "She refused to come downstairs."

My grandfather squinted at the film, searching for any abnormalities. He gripped a half-smoked cigar in one hand. "I wonder how she'll do when we have to take her over to surgery. I don't see anything out of the ordinary. Let Seichrest review the X-ray when he comes down later this week." He chomped on his cigar. "Your father said you did pretty well with those retractors yesterday. Maybe you could help me in surgery sometime?"

I fought back a smile and pulled down Edna Thorne's chest X-ray. "I'd like that."

Leaving his office, I bumped into Lowell Middleton. Mr. Middleton was a member of the hospital's board of directors and one of Waxahachie's leading citizens. The owner of one of the busiest car dealerships, Lowell Middleton, commanded a great deal of influence around our small town. He was boisterous and outspoken and had as many critics as supporters.

"Robbie, is that you?" Mr. Middleton asked. "My, how you've grown since I've seen you." He didn't wait for my reply and ducked into my grandfather's office. "W. C.," I heard him say, through the partially closed door, "we've got to talk."

I hung around outside the door.

"I've heard rumors," Middleton said, "that, ah . . . well, let me put it another way. We have a good community here. Everybody seems to know their place. When you wanted to build the Annex out back, the rest of the board and I went along. We did it because it was the right thing to do."

"Lowell, get to your point. I have patients to round on."

"It's not that I don't think Negroes are entitled to good health care. They are. Hell, I've got one working for me at home. I got four down at the dealership. Hard workers, all of them. What I mean to say is, they're like family to me." Middleton cleared his throat. "But here's the thing. These people are more comfortable with their own kind. Listen, I've been a big supporter of this hospital since we settled here. You delivered my granddaughter up on the third floor. You remember that? There're a lot of good folks around town getting nervous, not that I'm one of them. They think you might be planning to move the Negroes into the hospital with us."

"Is that such a terrible idea?"

"Tell me that's not what you're thinking."

"What's so wrong with putting all the sick people under one roof?"

"It'll never happen, W. C."

"See you at the next board meeting, Lowell," my grandfather said as he yanked open the door and strode past me. My grandfather hesitated at the outer door.

Lowell Middleton left the office the way he came, in a hurry. He stopped in the waiting area and turned to face my grandfather, his jaw fixed. "Dallas is only thirty miles up the road. From what I hear, they have some good hospitals up there, too. You don't watch yourself, and people around here might start making the drive."

After Lowell Middleton made his departure, my grandfather stood in the doorway looking at me. "I've seen a lot of things while working at this hospital. Sometimes you see the very best it has to offer. Sometimes you see the worst."

PART TWO

MORE THAN THE MEDICINES

10

DEFENSIVE MEDICINE

In the years since I last worked at the hospital, my life had changed in many ways. That summer before my junior year in high school, I fell in love. She was an incoming freshman with a long, blonde ponytail and two dimples. Her name was Janet. We dated for almost two years. When she realized how immature I was, she broke it off. My father encouraged me to enroll in a small liberal arts college back East. After almost failing out the second semester of my sophomore year, I had an epiphany about my future. I moved out of the fraternity house and into an apartment by myself. It worked. I turned things around, and got accepted into medical school. At the same time, I won back my high school sweetheart with the long, blonde ponytail and two dimples.

In the late fall of 1963, I got my letter of acceptance to medical school. There had been moments in college when I had doubts about a career in medicine. To cover my bets, I'd switched majors from science to mathematics. In the end, I realized that I wanted to be a part of the medical family. That desire kept calling me back to my father and grandfather and to the profession they had chosen.

A lot had changed at the hospital. A new maternity wing had been added. The operating and emergency rooms had been expanded into a suite of rooms. My grandfather had closed the Annex and now used the building for storage. Discrimination finally ended at our hospital and, as predicted, some of the good citizens of Waxahachie, along with Lowell Middleton, transferred their care to Dallas some thirty miles up the road. The irony was that the hospitals in Dallas had abandoned separate facilities for Negroes and whites years earlier.

I saw my grandfather in two roles. Away from the hospital, he was an unassuming man, often taking a backseat to the rest of the family. At the hospital, he was more of a benevolent dictator. When he spoke, everyone listened. That even included Oma Jones, who didn't normally listen to anybody but her pet parrot.

I stood in the office reception area, waiting.

"Your grandfather is ready to see you," Mrs. Smith, his nurse, said and then went back to her typewriter.

When I entered his office, my grandfather spoke first. "Did you read this?" He gestured at an article in the newspaper spread out on his desk. "If Congress passes this legislation, they'll end up telling us how we should take care of our patients."

"What legislation?"

"Since you're now going to be a doctor, I thought you might have been following this."

"I'm not sure what you're talking about." I looked over his shoulder and scanned the article.

The issue was a new government program called Medicare and how the new program would pay for health care for the elderly. The spokesman for the proposed legislation claimed Medicare would benefit both doctors and hospitals by helping them collect on services that had previously gone unfunded. Medicare was similar to the state-administered, federal Medicaid program for individuals and families with low incomes. Supporters of Medicare assured readers the new program would not interfere with decisions of health care delivery.

"Doesn't sound so bad to me," I said. "Says here, the government won't tell doctors how to practice medicine." I pointed to the final paragraph in the article. "If it goes through, you and the hospital will finally get paid for services you've written off for years."

"Despite what the bureaucrats in Washington think, the federal government does only two things better than the private sector: conduct war and collect taxes."

In the past, my grandfather had not been vocal about his political feelings. But the government's move into covering health care services had him riled.

"Washington doesn't pay for anything without strings," he said. He held his half-chewed stogie in his hand and waved it for emphasis. "Once the bureaucrats get their foot in the door, it's only a matter of time until they'll be telling us how much we can charge and finally what we can do."

"Do you really think this country would allow socialized medicine? My premed-student friends said it'd never happen. Doctors in this country wouldn't allow the government, or anyone else, to come in and tell them how to take care of patients."

"I'd like to think that's true."

"My father told me Dr. Leiber and his pals have been stirring up rumors about starting a new hospital." Dr. Leiber was an internist who moved to Waxahachie about five years ago.

"They'll never do it." My grandfather grumbled, then looked back at the papers on his desk. It was his way of letting me know that our meeting was at a close.

"See you Sunday at our house for lunch?" I asked.

He nodded. "Oh, Robbie. Congratulations."

Finally, my grandfather had given me his acknowledgment. I wasn't sure if he was congratulating me for acceptance to medical school or because I was getting married. As few compliments as he handed out, I guess it didn't matter.

I caught up with my father as he pulled the door closed to Maylene Neeley's room.

"Is she still calling you at all hours of the night?" I asked. Maylene owned the Forreston telephone company.

"Oh, yes. But, this time she might have something serious."

We ambled to the nurses' station. He grabbed Maylene's chart off the rack. "We'll talk more on the ride home."

He wasn't his usual self. In the car, I asked, "What's wrong?"

He pushed the old Buick faster, stirring up a plume of dust.

"Nothing. It's just been a hard week. Lots of really sick people, possibly including Maylene."

"That's nothing new. You've always had lots of sick people. Maybe you're just getting older?"

He eased off the accelerator. "Maybe it's just that I'm not able to adjust to changes the way I used to."

"Changes in what?" My curiosity was aroused.

We pulled up the grassy alley that led to our house, but my father made no attempt to get out. He said, "One of the most satisfying things about being a doctor was that people trusted me. No matter what the outcome, they knew I had done my best. And whatever happened, happened."

"What do you mean by was?"

"I'm being sued." His face was drawn. "Claims I missed the diagnosis of cancer."

My chest tightened at the news. Although we had often talked about the possibility of legal action against him, I thought the only doctors who got sued were the ones who took poor care of their patients. I never thought it was possible that my father could do anything wrong.

"Did the patient die?"

"No. She's going to live."

"What's the problem? You missed the diagnosis, but it was picked up in time. I can understand why she would be upset, but why sue?"

"I operated on her two years ago and found what we thought were metastatic tumors all over the inside of her abdomen. So your grandfather and I closed her back up and sent her to Dallas for chemotherapy."

"So she's cured of her cancer. Why is she suing?"

"Because now she's decided she never had cancer in the first place. Says we put her through two years of hell, along with the side-effects from the chemo." He looked over at me, a slight crack noticeable in his voice. "It's not that I want her to have cancer, but . . ."

"I don't see that her lawyer has a case. The pathology report will prove her wrong."

"We didn't get one. We thought the diagnosis looked so obvious. In retrospect, we made the wrong decision not to do a biopsy. But that's what the practice of medicine is all about, making the best decision with the facts you have available. I guess that's what bothers me the most, knowing that for the rest of my time in medicine, I will order extra laboratory tests and ask for unnecessary consultations just to protect myself in case I get sued."

"Isn't it possible she really had cancer and the chemotherapy cured her? Or what if, like Oral Roberts claims on his television ministry, she had a miracle?"

He swung open the door and dropped his feet to the ground. "Malpractice attorneys don't believe in miracles."

As the lawsuit dragged on and the initial shock wore off, we all fell back into our routines. My grandfather tended his patients. My father was busy in surgery. Janet and I made plans for the wedding.

"We set the date," I announced to Dorothy, my father's secretary, as I bounded into his outer office. I had thirty minutes before meeting my fiancée for lunch, and I was eager to share the good news. "June twentieth. I'm a lucky guy." With only two days left in my Christmas break, Janet had agreed to marry me. It would take a sacrifice on both our parts, and we would have to delay starting our family. Although the idea of being able to carry on the family name in medicine filled me with excitement, I had doubts that I would be able to live up to my father's and grandfather's expectations. Now I would ask another to join me in that journey, someone special who put her hopes in my hands.

Dorothy said, "You're going to invite me to the wedding?"

"You're at the top of my list. Where's my father?" I didn't usually bother him when he was seeing patients, but I thought a little father/son time was in order before I left for school.

"He's with Mrs. Cheetam in Room One, taking off some of her moles, and then it looks like he's through."

I moved on down the hall toward his office to wait. Stopping briefly in front of the partially closed door to Room One, I could hear the familiar sound of my father's humming. It reminded me of the metronome that sat atop the piano, ticking away, during those forced practice sessions when I was a kid. The instrument stood as a model of order, bringing a sense of calm and predictability to my failed music career after eight years of lessons.

I secluded myself in the far corner of his office with a two-month old *Life* magazine that I had lifted from the waiting room. Less than ten minutes passed when a piercing scream came from Room One.

I jumped to my feet and headed toward the exam room. As I approached, I heard sounds of thrashing and some garbled grunts and groans. Throwing open the door, I saw my father struggling to push Mrs. Cheetam, her eyes rolled up, back onto the examination table.

"What the hell?" I said.

"Are you just going to stand there?"

I rushed forward as the two of us were able to reposition Mrs. Cheetam's flailing body back onto the table.

Her eyes sprang open and she looked up at me. "Who are you?" My father was now propped up against the wall trying to catch his breath. "Oh Dr. Mayo, I'm so sorry. The last thing I remember was when you stopped humming. It nearly scared me to death."

After Mrs. Cheetam had gone home, I asked my father, "Are you okay?"

He nodded. We made our way back to his office, but I could tell he was shaken.

"After she started to fall off the table," he said, "all I could think of was having to face another lawsuit."

"How's the suit going?" I asked.

"The people from Medical Protective put me in touch with a big firm in Dallas. I talked to a new associate who specializes in these types of cases. He just moved here from California, where he says getting sued is a way of life."

"What did he tell you to do?"

"Let them make the next move. He said the patient has a pretty good case against us because we didn't do a biopsy."

"What about all the years of experience you and Pa have? Doesn't that count?"

"He said juries don't care about reputation and years of experience. All they see is a defenseless patient being exploited by some money-grabbing doctor."

"It may be that way in California, but not here."

"It's sad, but even if the patient wins, they are often left with very little after their lawyers get paid. According to the insurance company's attorney, my generation has not come into the twentieth century. He says that thinking of every patient as someone who might sue is the only way doctors in the future can protect themselves from losing everything they've worked for."

"She won't win," I said.

"Her lawyer has filed a suit against me for a hundred thousand dollars more than my malpractice insurance covers. So if he can convince the jury, we could be in real trouble. That's why the insurance agency suggested I settle before the suit goes much further."

"What about the principle of standing by your medical decision?"

"Principles won't put food on your plate." The characteristic assurance in his voice had vanished. This was the first time I had ever seen my father back down from a challenge, and it was not an image I admired. "I feel like I'm being held hostage. Not only am I at risk, but so is our family. The real tragedy is that patients will become our enemies."

"Will there ever come a time when doctors might move away from states like California, so they'll be less likely to be sued?"

He drew in a deep breath. "That would be a sad day indeed."

I felt bad leaving my father with such a burden, but it was time for me to leave for the airport in Dallas. The twin-engine prop plane that would carry me back to Pennsylvania was cramped and noisy. The idea of two months away from Janet and my upcoming exams left me wanting to be alone, so I chose a window seat in the last row and hoped for some measure of isolation. It didn't work out that way.

The woman next to me looked over at my organic chemistry book and said, "Are you going to be a doctor?" She was neatly dressed with prematurely graying hair. We made introductions, and I told her I was entering medical school the following fall. She said, "I'm a nurse or, at least, I was."

"Did you retire?"

"Not exactly. I've been in nursing for over sixteen years. My mother was, and my sister is now. But lately, things have begun to change. At my hospital, they're replacing many of us with aides to do the bedside care. The administrator claims that with rising costs, they can't afford to hire fully trained nurses the way they had before. For almost a year, about all I've done is pass out pills and fill out paperwork. They could hire a robot to do that. I guess they keep me on because the hospital needs that RN degree at the end of my name. It's for their accreditation."

"You mean the only time you work with patients is when you give them their medicines?"

The engines blunted her words. "Essentially. I meet the patients when they're admitted, and then again if there's an emergency. That's if I'm not tied up in meetings." She peered across me as the Dallas skyline began to fade in the distance. "Some of my friends in nursing are thinking about moving into administration. The pay and the chance of advancement are better. I'm going up to look around in Hartford, Connecticut. They tell me several of the large insurance companies are thinking about getting into health care coverage, like Blue Cross here in Texas."

"So, you're applying to work in the infirmary?"

"I'll probably be reviewing medical records."

I remembered how Mrs. McAndrews, our nurse in high school, would review the medical form my mother filled out at the start of each year if I was ever sent to her office with a problem.

"So you would evaluate patients' records to see if they need to see a doctor?"

She shook her head. "I would make recommendations on how much the company should pay for a particular medical service, or maybe if a particular service should even be covered at all."

"My father calls that socialized medicine. Instead of the government telling doctors how to practice medicine, it would be insurance companies."

"These companies have a responsibility to their stockholders to manage their resources." Her voice grew louder. "With all the new tests and treatments, there's going to be a lot more money spent on medical care. The potential for a lot more profit, too. So if the insurance companies become involved, it only seems reasonable they should have a say in how their money is spent."

"Please don't take this wrong, but why do you think an insurance company would use a nurse to make those decisions instead of a doctor?"

"Because I'll charge less."

With the roar of the engines around me, I settled back in my seat. I looked out the window and realized, *I'm not in Waxahachie anymore.*

11

MY GRANDFATHER'S GREATEST GIFT

My father said into the phone, "There have been grumblings for the last several months, but I never thought Dr. Leiber and his associates were serious. Not until this morning. So I felt you should be warned before you get home."

My father's unexpected, late-evening telephone call had interrupted my studying marathon before diving into two straight days of final exams. He had hinted there might be a problem when I was home for Christmas, but my grandfather had shrugged it off. Now, it appeared the doctors' rebellion against my grandfather wasn't just a rumor.

With Janet at the University of Texas in Austin, I felt as if I was studying for two people. I still paid my dues to the fraternity, though my involvement was virtually over. When I wasn't in class, I stayed holed up in my one-room apartment, only retreating to a neighborhood diner across the street for meals and brief moments of conversation with a couple of classmates who lived in the apartment below me. My success and my upcoming life with Janet depended on how well I did on these exams. My father was counting on me to come home with a diploma. I knew his call was important, but the timing couldn't have been worse.

I found it difficult to believe that the group of doctors would really go so far as to build a new hospital. I said, "Maybe they're just bluffing."

"Dorothy knows somebody down at the county commissioner's office. She claims they've already filed for a building permit."

"So they're ready to break ground?"

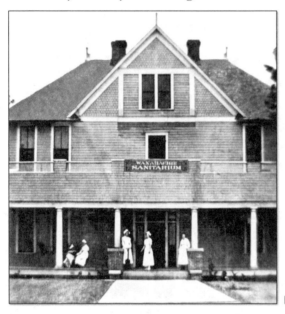

| Original Waxahachie Sanitarium

My grandfather's command of the hospital had been a bone of contention for some time with this group of physicians that had settled in our town about five years ago.

My grandfather's history with the hospital was well known. At the end of World War I, he had converted an old boarding house into Waxahachie's first hospital. He then personally guaranteed the sale of city bonds necessary to construct the new building in the late 1920s. Dr. W. C. had been considered the patriarch of medicine in our little community for the last fifty years. His medical peers never openly contested his position as both chief of staff and administrator-in-residence. I never really knew why they didn't. I suspected they were afraid that if they were caught complaining too loudly, he would dump some of the administrative responsibility on their shoulders. Due to the nature of their largely rural practices, they were not prepared or willing to handle the burden.

With the arrival of Dr. Ryan Leiber and two associates he brought in a year later, that attitude had changed. They wanted to participate, and they wanted a whole new system of administration. And they were committed to building a separate facility across town, if they didn't get their way. Even though publicly they heaped praise on my grandfather for his accomplishments, they privately declared that the days of his autocratic governance had to end. I found their approach callous, but wondered if I might not feel the same way if I were in their situation. As a gesture of good faith, the doctors were saying my grandfather would be allowed to keep his office on the second floor. But his input to the institution he had birthed almost a half a century before would be no more than that of any other doctor who admitted patients to the hospital.

"I was there when Leiber handed him the letter this morning," my father said. "We all knew that someday it would have to change around here. I'd hoped your grandfather would retire by then. A dagger to his throat would not hurt him more."

"What did Pa say?"

"Nothing. Absolutely nothing. He just shoved the letter in his pocket and headed to surgery."

"Where is he now?"

"The last I saw of him, he'd loaded up his golf clubs and was heading over to Dr. Hawkins' office."

Only a miracle could avoid the looming crisis between Dr. Leiber and my grandfather. But miracles do happen: I passed my finals.

▬ ▪ ▬

In the four years I'd spent on the East Coast, I had developed a close bond to the region and its people. Despite being born in New York City while my father completed his surgery residency, I was a Texan through and through. It was time to return home and start the long and arduous journey of becoming a doctor. With my car crammed to the roof, I began the long drive back from college. The hours of solitude gave me time to contemplate what I would encounter in the weeks ahead. How would my grandfather respond to Leiber's demands? How would I make it through the wedding festivities?

My car moved steadily ahead on the interstate.

With Dr. Leiber, the government, and the insurance companies all fighting for control, what would the practice of medicine be like for my generation? How would I handle the death of my first patient? My first lawsuit? My uncertainties were not limited just to my life as a physician, but also to my role as a husband and a father. I had chosen for a mate a woman about whom I had no uncertainties at all. But would I be able to fulfill my obligations to the family we would be starting? The ballet recitals? The soccer games? The open houses at school? The seemingly small choices that made the difference between personal success and failure. Following in the footsteps of my father and grandfather would take a monumental effort. To be the husband and father I wanted to be would take more. I had come to realize that life was about priorities. My values were my choice, and how I applied those values would be the measure of how I would be remembered.

While I was pondering my legacy, my grandfather was busy living his.

He abruptly resigned as administrator of the hospital. His decision caught the family by surprise. When my grandfather made up his mind, he always acted fast. As we waited for him to arrive for lunch for the Sunday family get together, we were all a little on edge.

"Avoid discussing the hospital situation," my mother said, "unless he brings it up." She set the silverware around the dining room table. "Tell him about your wedding plans instead."

When my grandfather walked in, I reached out to greet him with a handshake. He returned my gesture with his usual limp two-finger clasp. He always claimed he was saving his hands for surgery, a quirk I had never been able to understand since he had held both the tennis and golf championships at the Country Club on numerous occasions.

I said, "All our wedding festivities are going to cut into your golf game."

"Looks like I'll have plenty of time now," he said. "You never liked golf much, did you?"

"I'm not any good at it."

"There's a lesson to be learned there," he said. He pointed his chewed-up stogie in my direction. "It's about putting forth the effort until you are good. For some that comes easier than for others. It says a lot about the kind of doctor you're going to turn out to be."

"I plan to work hard in medical school," I said.

"It takes a lifetime commitment. At least, I thought it did." His eyes suddenly turned sad.

"What do you mean?"

"Medicine has been my life. Golf and tennis are just distractions that help me keep the other in perspective. Your father claimed he wanted to be an actor, but I prodded him into being a doctor. I wanted to be a professional tennis player. Those are dreams. This is reality. I've always felt we needed to do something with our lives that makes a difference. Many of these physicians coming out today think differently. They put a much higher priority on being with their family and their pleasures than those of us who came here in the early part of the century. When I'm told the average life expectancy for a general practitioner in rural Texas is around fifty, I'm not sure these young doctors are wrong. The irony is . . ."

Just then my mother called us to lunch. "Do you want to talk about this later?" I asked.

He nodded.

After lunch, in the relative isolation of the den, I decided to ask about his resignation.

"Why did you do it?"

"Because, if I hadn't, they would have built another hospital, and Waxahachie would have been split. I couldn't have done that, not to the patients who have depended on me for the last fifty years." He looked off across the room. "At first, I was resentful, took it personally, but they're probably right. Medicine is becoming a big business. If this hospital is going to stay in the black, we need to bring in one of those executive types who is experienced in finance."

"So what now?"

"I've still got my practice, and . . ." His eyes shifted uneasily, as if he were holding something back. "You'll read about it in the paper tomorrow anyway. I also gave them the laboratory and X-ray facilities, plus the two hundred and twenty-five thousand dollars from those accounts I had set aside."

"Set aside for what?"

"I guess some of us who lived through the hard times never got over the lessons of the Great Depression. The money really wasn't mine anyway. It belonged to the patients who supported this hospital."

In the stock market crash of 1929, my father told me, my grandfather had pledged his own money to keep the bank open. I wondered if he hadn't already done enough.

"What about your retirement?"

"I've got enough to get me by. When I'm gone, there's only one thing I can leave behind to my family of any real value." Digging into his pants pocket, he deposited the contents on the cushion beside me. Then stood up and slowly made his way out of the room.

I picked up the shiny object on the seat cushion—a gold Zippo lighter. I rolled the cigarette lighter over until my eyes locked onto the engraving on the other side: the six letters of our family name.

My grandfather's resignation and generous gift to the community made the headlines of our newspaper. Soon after, the board of trustees voted to rename the hospital after him. My family and I attended the dedication ceremony. Although my grandfather tried to share much of the credit for pioneering modern medicine in and around Waxahachie, the honor fell mostly on his shoulders. The behind-the-scene rumblings that led to his departure were still known only to a few. And that's how he wanted it.

"No need to dwell in the past," he whispered in my ear. I stood behind him at the ceremony. "Any baggage you carry only slows you down."

I beamed with pride, looking out over the sparse crowd of hospital employees and devoted citizens who had braved the inclement weather for the unveiling. The representative from the hospital removed the cloth from the new sign. My heart jumped, seeing it for the first time. I tucked the wrinkled program under my arm, reached in my pocket and pulled out the Zippo lighter. I understood that the family name was his ultimate gift. What we did with it in the future was up to us.

12

BEING A DOCTA'

My father delivered the news in the matter of fact way he delivered all bad news: he was in the advanced stages of emphysema. I grabbed for the chair in front of his desk and tumbled into it. I didn't know what to say. Well into my second year of medical school, I'd begun to look forward to beginning my practice. Nonetheless, I had reservations about returning home as the number three general surgeon in the family. I dreaded the thought of constantly being compared to Dr. W. C. and Dr. Mayo. With this diagnosis, the possibility of working alongside my father evaporated.

He shook his head. "I should have taken my own advice and quit smoking years ago. I've been fighting this dependency almost all my life."

"Who else knows?"

"About the smoking? Dorothy walked in on me a time or two." He sounded grim. "Sometimes I even send her out for a pack, since I'm afraid for anyone else to know."

"Can't you be treated?" After a year and a half of medical school, I was familiar with only the rudiments of the degenerative disease of the lungs.

"They can treat the problems as they arise and give me oxygen when I need it. Once the disease gets to a certain stage there's no turning it around, even if I stop smoking."

"I thought you had stopped," I said.

He pulled open his desk drawer and grabbed a small metallic inhaler. After sucking in two quick blasts, he looked at me, making no attempt to answer.

"Why?" I asked.

"Please don't tell your mother." His head bowed. "I'd promised her I'd quit, but I just couldn't."

My father had carried my mother's engagement ring in his pocket for a year and a half before she accepted it. When he first saw her picture, she'd been dating his medical school roommate in Boston. My father predicted they would marry when he first saw her picture. After several years of courtship, he won her heart. Then only a brief two years after their wedding, and my arrival on the scene, came World War II. They were forced into a three-year separation, with my mother and me dividing our time between his parents in Waxahachie and her mother on the East Coast, while my father plied the tools of his profession on the European front. I knew my father felt that after all her years of loyalty to him, my mother deserved better than spending the last part of her life with an invalid.

"Shouldn't you tell her?"

"I love your mother. But this is something I have to face alone."

"She can help you, you know. Hiding the problem is only going to hurt her more when she finds out."

"It's my demon."

Even amid my sympathy and pain for him, I felt betrayed. How could he do this to me? How could he knowingly cut short his life when I needed his continuing advice for making important decisions about my future? What about my sister and my mother? Then I realized my concerns were all about us—what we wanted from him, not what he needed from those who loved him.

"She's going to find out."

"Soon enough." He pushed back from his desk, his labored breathing ameliorated by the effects of the medication. "Maybe I can give her a couple more good years before she has to know." He rose to his feet. "Since you're about to go into the clinics, I knew you couldn't be fooled much longer."

He had entrusted me with the knowledge of his illness not as his son, but as a future physician. My role in the time he had remaining had become very important to him. On that day, he taught me something crucial about being a doctor: never betray the confidences of one's patients.

My father had unknowingly become my second patient, after Connie the rabbit.

"Do you want to tag along while I make rounds?" he asked.

I nodded. There was nothing more to say.

Our first stop was the nurses' station. Nurse Delmer said, "You're going to make a fine doctor someday. Just like your father."

I smiled, always a little ill at ease knowing that everyone in our little community took for granted I would just sail through my medical training because my father and grandfather were doctors. The first year and a half of medical school had been a bitch. The inner workings of humans were far more complex than those of frogs and nematodes.

I said, "I start on the wards next week with live patients."

"He can't wait for you to come back and join him." Mrs. Delmer grabbed a clipboard with the list of patients and scooted along after my father.

Picking up the pace just behind her, I said, "That won't happen for quite a while."

Our next stop was Mrs. Snider. My father pushed through the door of her room. "Well, Mrs. Snider, how're you feeling today?"

The woman rustled in her bed. "Oh, Dr. Mayo, I hurt so bad." Her pale face was greased with perspiration. "I just don't know if I'm going to make it."

"Sure you will. The day after surgery is always the worst."

"You told me that yesterday. My surgery was two days ago."

"Well, that just proves some folks take a little longer to heal than others." He looked over at the clipboard Mrs. Delmer was holding. "Are her vitals okay?"

She nodded. "Temp ninety-nine point six, blood pressure a hundred twenty-four over . . ." Her voice trailed off as my father turned back to the patient.

Then I first noticed a large white porcelain jar under Mrs. Snider's bed. Bending over to get a better look, I saw it was filled with a dark brown syrupy substance. I assumed it was drainage from her surgical wound site, but looking closer, I saw no tube coming down from her bed. "What's that?" I asked my father.

"Black-strap molasses. Mrs. Snider brought it with her from home," he said. "Putting it under her bed is a remedy for arthritis that's been in her family for generations."

When we reached the hallway, I said, "Molasses won't help her arthritis."

"Are you sure?"

"They don't talk about it in the textbooks."

"Maybe not, but it's not going to hurt. What matters is what she thinks. Sometimes these home remedies, mixed with a little compassion, are the most valuable medicines we can offer."

———— ■ ————

In the year that followed, the lawsuit against my father dragged on. His lawyer wanted to take the case to court. His strategy was that the jurors were more likely to believe in miraculous healing. My father and the insurance agency weren't so sure.

In that same long year, lots of things changed. Dr. Sturgess, author of the misleading newspaper ads, moved on before he ever started a practice in Waxahachie. Several former patients in Houston were looking for a piece of his hide, and our little town must not have been far enough away.

Dr. Leiber got his way and was elected the first chief of staff of the hospital. His first order of business was to put together a search committee for an administrator to run the business of the hospital, a move that even my father agreed should have happened years sooner. In a gesture of goodwill, Dr. Leiber and the other doctors on staff elected my father secretary-treasurer, a position he accepted with his usual graciousness.

On my next visit home, I pulled into the hospital parking lot. I wanted to say a quick hello to Ruby Profett, Lenny Pope, and my father if he was around. It started to sprinkle when a thunderclap boomed off in the distance. Dashing from my car, I spotted Gene outside the door to the hospital's emergency entrance.

I said, "Looks like it's going to be a downpour."

"We could sure use it," Gene said, a plume of smoke from his pipe quickly dispersed in the wind. "I've been having to water my garden. Runs up the bills pretty quick, you know. If we don't get some help soon, I'd be better off buying my vegetables at the store." He let his pipe slip from his lips to his hands. "Your father and your grandfather sure are proud of you. They just struts around here, talking about what all you've been doing down there in Galveston gettin' your medical education and everything."

"I'm only starting my third year. I've got a long way to go until I'm a doctor."

"A docta'." Gene looked over at me as the first droplets of rain splashed across his shoulder. "You know I've been around here working alongside your grandfather since I was about your age." He stepped back, shielding himself from the increasing rain. "I've seen a lot of them come and go here at this hospital. Some of them pretty good and some of them, let's say, not as good as they think they are. I had a cousin up in Dallas who was real sick. In fact, he was all eat up with cancer. The doctors in that big hospital over on Gaston Avenue said there was nothing more they could do for him, so they sent him home with a bottle of pain pills to die. All his folks had either passed or moved on. He was scared. Scared not so much of dying, but being alone when he died. So I brought him down here to my house, and your grandfather came out and looked him over."

The rain pelted down inches beyond our reach.

"So what happened?" I asked.

"He agreed my cousin didn't have no chance of livin' and what the doctors at that Gaston Avenue hospital had done was right and proper. So we just kept giving him those pills until he was no longer conscious." Gene looked off toward the Annex. "But what I was leadin' to was your grandfather came out every day until my cousin died. Most of the time he didn't do nothin' except maybe bring him more pills, but the important thing, my cousin knew he was there."

"That wouldn't happen today." I was confident that the advances in surgery and treatment for cancer would have prolonged Gene's cousin's life. "In Houston, they've got this whole hospital set aside for treating cancer."

"Do they cure them all?" he asked.

"Not all of them."

"What do they do for those who ain't cured?"

I said nothing.

"You see, it's not much different from when my cousin died. Except maybe the doctors save a few more and keep the rest alive for a while longer." Gene turned away from the storm as if to head back inside. "What your grandfather did for my cousin didn't come from that bottle of pills. It came from here." He lowered the mouthpiece of his pipe and pointed to his left breast pocket. "Being a docta' is not just about what you know. It's about what you feel."

13

SETTING PRIORITIES

M y father called and said my grandfather had died. I was
shocked. My grandfather and I didn't communicate easily.
Nonetheless, the influence he had on me was incalculable. I
choked back tears, realizing he wouldn't be there for my graduation from
medical school. I loved him as any boy does his grandfather. Stronger
than my love was my admiration for what he'd accomplished.

"What happened?" I asked.

"When your grandfather woke up from surgery, the doctor told him it
was cancer. Then he closed his eyes and never opened them."

The week before, my grandfather had noted bleeding from his rectum.
According to my father, he checked into Baylor Hospital. Exploratory
surgery revealed he had a localized carcinoma of the colon. The surgeon
felt he had been able to remove all the tumor.

My grandfather had a dark secret very few people knew about, one I
would only discover after his death: he had a pathologic fear of dying
from cancer.

At the memorial service, my father and I spoke briefly about it.

"I think it was because he saw so many of his patients suffer," he said.
"Your grandfather once told me it took away their dignity. After he got the
news, my guess is he just decided to go back to sleep rather than lose his."

I had always thought of my grandfather as immortal. Here he was struck down by one of the maladies he had dedicated his life to conquer. What I felt was more an emptiness, an end to a relationship that never quite came to fruition. More than anything, I wanted him to see me become a doctor.

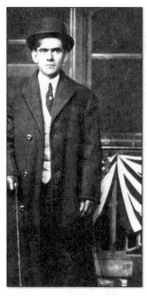

| Dr. W. C.

After the memorial service, friends and family crammed into my grandfather's home. Every couch and chair was occupied. Well-wishers even sat on the arms of his over-stuffed sofa, any place they could rest their bodies while they filled their stomachs.

"He was a good man," one dark-haired cousin mumbled to the group.

This cousin, his plate laden with casserole and two pieces of homemade banana-nut bread, kept droning repeated inferences about my grandfather's will. "When our folks traveled from Tennessee to Texas, we had nothing but each other. I sure hope Bill didn't forget those times. We've worked hard for what we got. Here we are sharing our grief once again. He was kin. We were close, is all I'm saying." He stopped momentarily to glance at my father.

"He gave it all away," my father answered with an expression of satisfaction on his face.

"Gave what away?"

"Except for this house and the property he bought his mother in Longview, it's all gone," my father said. "He said the money came from the community. It was only right that it go back."

"What about us. What about his family?" The man frowned. "Did he want us to get nothing? I mean, didn't he want us to have something to remember him by?"

"He did," my father said and then he stood and walked from the room. I'll never know exactly what he meant, but I think my father was referring to my grandfather's good name. He left it emblazoned on the face of the hospital. I fingered the engraving of his initials on the Zippo lighter in my pocket.

The funeral had drained my family. Janet and I elected to extend our stay in Waxahachie an extra day so she could see her family.

That night, we sat around the kitchen table making small talk. It must have been close to seven when an ambulance stopped outside our house. My mother answered the door and after a hushed conversation raced into the kitchen. "It's Buddy, the ambulance driver," my mother said. She stared at my father. "There's been an accident at the gin, and they need you to get down there now. A worker has his arm caught in the stripping machine."

"I'll have to run by the hospital and pick up a set of instruments," my father said. He shoved away from the table and headed for the front door. "All I've got here are the medicines in my bag."

Seeing the shock on Janet's face, I realized this was her first real exposure to life as part of a family of doctors. I pecked her on the cheek for reassurance and then grabbed my father's medical bag by the back door.

Outside, Buddy shouted at my father. "Dr. Mayo, this guy at the gin, he's got his arm trapped up to his shoulder. If you don't do something quick, he's gonna die."

My father grabbed his medical bag from my hand. "If we have to amputate, we'll need more than we've got here."

"I'm way ahead of you." Buddy signaled for my father to follow him to the waiting ambulance. "I sent Mike over to the hospital in the other ambulance to pick up a surgical set-up tray and your amputation knives, just in case. He should be over at the gin before we get there."

Buddy's driving partner, Mike Wiegal, was a legend in Waxahachie. Mike was a closet race car driver, and no one would ever deny he was good at what he did. He'd probably saved a few lives along the way.

By the time we arrived at the gin, Mike was there with my father's instruments. "Here you go, Doc." He thrust forward the two packages wrapped in sterile white towels.

From inside the cotton gin's corrugated metal walls came a shrill cry of pain.

"He's hurtin' real bad," Buddy muttered.

My father disappeared into the building. I followed close behind.

Cotton gins all have a familiar smell, somewhere between musty old clothes and boiling black-strap molasses. He pushed through the small crowd of onlookers.

"Let's make some room here."

The space opened around a large machine that stripped cotton fiber from the seed. Halfway up the conveyor belt dangled a man, his torn shirt soaked in blood, his arm suspended over his head between the hooked teeth of this ghostly contraption.

"Please, Doc." The man's voice was a whisper. "Do something."

"Put this thing in reverse," my father shouted.

"She only goes one way, Doc. It's either off or on," a voice in the crowd said.

"What about taking this thing apart to get his arm out?"

The large room stood in silence as the machine's operator stepped forward. "Doc, it'd take two hours to disassemble this thing and get Crutcher out, maybe an hour and a half if we're lucky."

"By then it'll be too late," my father said. "What you get out of there may be so chewed up, it won't be worth saving. Robbie, draw me up a cc of morphine."

I pulled out a sterile needle and syringe and a small brown bottle labeled morphine sulfate. By the time I drew up the medicine, my father had already checked the tightness of the makeshift tourniquet wrapped around Crutcher's mangled arm.

"Get a vein on his other arm," he shouted out to me. He reached up once again to finger the knotted belt wound tightly just below the mangled flesh.

I retrieved the thin rubber strap from his bag and wrapped it tightly around Crutcher's other arm about six inches above his elbow.

"I found a vein," I said.

"See if you can give him the morphine while I set up here." He signaled to Mike, who moved forward to lay the two sterile trays on the conveyor belt just below Crutcher's dangling feet. My father's eyes moved back up to Crutcher. "I don't see we have any other choice, son."

I was able to get the needle into the vein on my first try. I held back injecting him until I got the word from my father. "Ready?" I asked.

He nodded and continued to unwrap the sterile instruments. I popped loose the rubber tourniquet and pushed on the plunger of the syringe until its contents disappeared into the now-collapsing vein. In thirty seconds, Crutcher's arm began to relax as the powerful pain-reliever found its mark deep within the receptors of his brain. My father laid out his instruments on the sterile drape.

"Pour some iodine over his arm right about there," he said.

Crutcher screamed when the scalpel pierced his skin. My father worked quickly, picking up a small saw to finish severing his arm.

"Buddy," my father called out, his hand still tightly clasped to the bloody stub of Crutcher's arm. "Get me some of those sterile towels over here, then let him down and move him onto the gurney so I can finish at the hospital."

I noticed anguish on my father's face. "What's wrong?" I asked in a low voice.

"Get me the nebulizer out of my coat. I left it in the ambulance."

I returned with my father's medicine.

"Asthma," my father said, inhaling two quick bursts off the small apparatus. "It's all this dust and cotton fibers."

Buddy stood over us, watching. "My brother had that problem too," he said. "Any little thing set him off. Then again, he smoked to the day he died."

At the hospital, my father cleaned and sutured Crutcher's arm and checked on him one more time before calling it a night.

On our way home, I told him I knew that what he went through at the cotton gin wasn't asthma.

He didn't say a word as we bumped over the gravel-topped road. When our house came into view, he said, "With your grandfather gone, I can't do this on my own." The lines on his face had now grown into ruts. "The way I see it, I don't have that much longer anyway."

I was about to say something when he stopped the car and sucked in one final puff from his nebulizer. He reached for the door-handle and looked back at me. "A specialist in Dallas said if I quit pushing myself, if I stay clear of people with colds, if . . . well, it gives me another five years."

"Five years for what?"

"You know what," he said with a hint of anger in his voice. "I put the word out I'm looking for a partner. What I need is someone who'll buy the practice and let me retire."

Now I was angry. "What about the smoking?"

"Haven't had one in over a week. But I'm afraid it's too little too late."

"It's never too late," I said. The weight of our conversation was more than I could take. I fought back tears. "Maybe your condition will stabilize. Maybe we can go on like we've been."

He stuffed the breathing device back in his pocket. "That would be nice. I could spend some time with your mother without worrying about the next telephone call. I might learn to let go of that tightness in my chest anytime I hear a siren." His eyes softened. "She deserves that as much as I do." His hand dropped away from the door handle. "When I first proposed to your mother, I asked her never to make me choose between her needs and my patients'. You know what? In over thirty-seven years of marriage, she never has."

14

GIVING UNCLE SAM HIS DUE

I spent my junior year of medical school working on the wards and in the clinics. The work made me feel like a real doctor. Our professors reminded us to tell our patients we were students. These people were so grateful to be attended by someone wearing a white smock that our status didn't matter. My reservations about not being up to the task grew dimmer as I took on more and more responsibility. Even in my brief tenure working at John Sealy Hospital in Galveston, I could already see the changes in medicine from my days at the Waxahachie hospital. As scientific advances grew, so did the

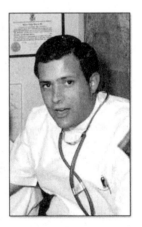

Rob Tenery, MD
Photographer: Janet Tenery

importance of the bottom line. The reason was that costs were rising. The latest tests and treatments were expensive, and someone had to foot the bill. If patients at John Sealy Hospital couldn't afford to pay, patients who once occupied the Annex certainly couldn't either.

Janet taught at the Catholic grade school, but her talk about starting a family had taken on a more serious note. It was only a matter of time until I took on the role as breadwinner. My internship, now only a year away, would pay me a small salary. We could make it as long as we stuck to our frugal ways.

I hoped the Vietnam war would be over by the time I finished my internship. Although President Nixon was winding down the United States presence in Vietnam, my class would likely be called to active duty. The draft was no longer in effect, but doctors were treated differently. The Berry Plan ensured that every male medical school graduate, with a few exceptions for National Guard service, was inducted into the military for a two-year hitch.

The president of my medical school in Galveston, Dr. Therman Becker, also moonlighted as a one-star general in the Texas National Guard. A plastic surgeon, he had helped pioneer one of the best reconstructive surgery programs in the country. A giant of a man, only his girth surpassed his confidence. He was reportedly the first surgeon to create an artificial vagina. The procedure was developed to help a young girl who had been badly disfigured in an accident. News of the operation was sensationalized, drawing a group of prospective patients who were unhappy with their birth gender. Beyond his medical renown, he also claimed to be best friends with the surgeon general of the United States. They had been stationed in the Pacific together during World War II.

Now in my final year of medical school, I'd changed my mind four times about my specialty. With my father and grandfather both general surgeons, the logical choice would have been to follow in their footsteps. Finally, I decided on plastic surgery. The reason I gave was that I did not want my efforts buried deep in the abdomen where no one could see them. Closer to the truth were the lingering doubts that I could ever live up to their reputations.

Janet and I had developed a strong affinity for Galveston. With Becker's respected program in my chosen area, the island community seemed like a perfect fit to continue my training. Unfortunately, Uncle Sam had other plans for me. Dr. Becker heard of my plight and called me in for a visit along with a fellow senior classmate, Alan Alton.

"You're Mayo's boy?" Dr. Becker said from behind his massive desk. Alan and I cowered in the over-sized chairs before him. "Good man.

Done a lot for the doctors of this state."

I nodded. Becker was referring to my father's recent stint as president of the state medical association. He had helped the university acquire its operating funds through the state legislature.

He said, "I hear you boys want to come back here and join my plastic surgery program?" Dr. Becker was famous for his one-sided conversations. "Good choice. You know, we were one of the first to create a . . ." He let the sentence hang. "We'll save that story for another time. You've probably heard I'm also a general in the National Guard." He leaned back in his chair, the buttons on his shirt stretched to the limit. "Just one well-placed call to my friend, the surgeon general, telling him you're my boys and your Berry Plan deferral should be as good as done."

"Thank you, Dr. Becker," I said.

His massive hand reached for the telephone atop his desk. "Consider it done."

Two weeks later my rejection arrived. No deferral. Alan's came the same day. When I laid the letter on Dr. Becker's desk, it was the only time I'd seen the man speechless.

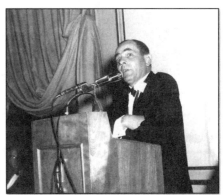

Dr. Mayo
Compliments of the Texas Medical Association

Before I was shipped off to war, I still had my internship to complete. Janet and I packed our belongings and headed to Dallas, where I had an internship position waiting at Parkland Hospital, the same hospital in which John F. Kennedy spent his final moments. During that year in Dallas, we tried unsuccessfully to have a baby. Soon thereafter, we adopted our son, Trey. Fortunately, the modest salary I earned as an intern allowed Janet to be a stay-at-home mom. Our luxuries were few. With me working over a hundred hours a week and the two of us taking care of a brand new baby, there wasn't much time for luxuries, anyway.

My orders from the U.S. Army were to begin basic training immediately after my internship. We were both concerned that I'd spend one year of my two-year obligation in Vietnam. My grandfather had served during World War I. My father was stationed at a four-hundred-bed Army evacuation hospital in France during World War II. As far as I was concerned, I was just following the family tradition.

Weeks later, along with 399 other physicians from around the country, we reported for duty at 0800 hours on July 21, 1969, to the giant orientation hall at Fort Sam Houston in San Antonio, Texas.

"Gentlemen," the officer said. He wore starched Army fatigues. "You are privileged to have been chosen to join the finest fighting machine the world has ever seen. You doctors have a choice about where you will be assigned in Vietnam."

From my limited experience, I'd never seen the word choice in print, much less thrown out in public. That term was used by the Air Force and even the Navy, but never the Army; that was, unless strings were attached, such as extending the recruit's tour of duty.

"Gentlemen, an aid-station is located 1,760 yards back from the front line, or one mile in civilian talk. We staff them with general medical officers, or GMOs. That's for those of you who don't have a designated specialty."

He was talking about me. And I knew that one mile was nothing for artillery shells.

"Those of you who are willing to avail yourself of one of the army's other choices will be assigned to one of our evacuation hospitals, which are located slightly over five thousand yards behind the front line. Even more attractive, you might join our Special Forces program, which also entitles you to an extra one hundred and fifty dollars a month in flight pay."

When the officer called for volunteers, I made my way to the Special Forces line.

"Lieutenant," the same officer said, "Just sign right here."

Picking up the clipboard with the military form attached, I reached for the pen when my eyes locked on the word *paratrooper.* "Sir, what does this mean?"

"It means, Lieutenant, that to qualify for the Special Forces program, you're going to have to make two jumps and two rappelings out of a helicopter."

My hand locked in its position. "You mean parachuting?"

He nodded.

Afraid of heights, I put down the unsigned form and quickly moved over to the line for anesthesia, since it was shorter than the one for orthopedics. I had never had a great deal of interest in either anesthesia or orthopedics. But to be an extra two miles away from the front line and not to have to jump out of a helicopter, I wasn't about to complain.

After basic training, I was promoted to captain and transferred to Fort Bragg in North Carolina. There I completed what I referred to as my "Heathkit residency" in anesthesiology in thirty-five days. I based the term on the self-assembly kit of the 1950s that ham radio operators used to put together their own transmitting equipment. My own inadequacy at anesthesia was repugnant to me. But this was war, and there was an acute shortage of orthopedic surgeons and anesthesiologists. The Army set up on-the-job training programs to fill this critical gap. We were supposed to work under the supervision of fully trained specialists. However, as President Nixon reduced the U.S. presence in the combat zone, the only physicians sent to Vietnam were replacements for those who came home early because of illness or injury. I was sent to Fort Benjamin Harrison in Indianapolis until I was needed in the war zone.

On the first day of my new assignment, I swung by the operating suite to get acquainted. That was when I saw the schedule for the next day's cases. Three surgeries were listed, all under my name.

The operating room supervisor and registered nurse, Lt. Col. Peaves, said, "First on your list is the general's wife. He's the head man on the base. John, being a nurse anesthetist and all, didn't want to do her, so we've been putting off her gallbladder surgery until you arrived. Way too much risk for his level of training."

John was a career-Army nurse anesthetist and infinitely more experienced than I was. "Where's John?" I asked.

"On leave. It started today," Peaves said. He turned toward the swinging doors that led to the sterile part of the operating room. "See you tomorrow, Captain."

I made a beeline to the hospital's commanding officer. I tapped on his partially open door. "Colonel." My palms sweated as I stood in front of Colonel Hale, the only career physician on the staff. "When I checked tomorrow's operating schedule, they have me down to do the anesthesia on General Golf's wife."

"Sit down, Captain. John's waited some time for you to arrive. He's due to have kidney surgery at Walter Reed."

"Yes sir. I understand. May I ask who else I'll be working with?"

The graying colonel, whose medical specialty was allergy, looked over from his cluttered desk. "You're it, son. You're not just the new chief of anesthesia. You have the operating room and recovery areas too. It's all yours."

"Colonel, I didn't do an anesthesia rotation in medical school or even during my internship. At Fort Bragg, I had only five weeks of training. I've never done an unassisted case."

The colonel removed his half-glasses and rubbed his temples. "I'm sure the Army thought you were well trained, or they wouldn't have sent you up here."

"You tell General Golf that, sir."

"Tell the general what, Captain?" Colonel Hale leaned forward in his chair, his cheeks flushed.

"About my experience, sir. That his wife will be my first unsupervised case after only five weeks of training. Sir!"

Colonel Hale eased back in his chair, stared at me for what seemed an eternity, and then reached over to the intercom. "Get General Golf on the phone for me," he bellowed.

Silence enveloped the room as seconds crawled into minutes. The only sounds were the colonel's fingers drumming on his desk. "He's on the line, sir," the secretary said.

"General. I understand your wife is scheduled for surgery at our hospital tomorrow. Although my doctors do an excellent job of taking care of our patients here on the base, I feel your wife deserves the very best the Army has to offer." The colonel spun around in his chair. "That's why I am putting in a request to have her transferred to Walter Reed Medical Center, sir."

I choked back my relief as the colonel finished his conversation with the general. "Thank you, sir," I forced out.

"Any other requests, Captain?"

Still unsure whether the colonel had acted because he was a doctor first or just didn't want the blot on his record in case the general's wife had a problem, I decided to put in my request for one more stipulation.

"No children. Sir. I'm not qualified. The University of Indiana Medical Center has an excellent pediatric hospital, and they're only twenty minutes away."

My first few surgeries went well. No one had a bad outcome because of something I did or didn't do. The operating room at Fort Benjamin Harrison averaged three to four cases a day. When I wasn't in surgery, I was farmed out to the outpatient clinic and covered the emergency room at night. All the physicians took turns. That was except for Colonel Hale, whom none of us trusted to take a call since he appeared more administrator than doctor.

A week into my stay, I was on night duty. A corpsman rushed up to my cot near the emergency room and shook me awake. "Captain," the corpsman said. "We have a patient who needs a doctor. He's a two-star general."

I glanced down at my watch. It was two forty-five in the morning.

"Did the general say what was wrong?"

"Sir, you don't ask generals anything. They tell you what they want."

Half-squinting in the light, I stumbled into the small examining room.

"General, what seems to be the problem?"

"Captain, I've got a bad back problem. Spasm from a war injury," he mumbled. The General was disheveled in a wrinkled Army jacket. "I need some Demerol to break the pain."

The man's oversized red nose and shaking hands told me there was more to the general's problem than a back spasm. "Sir, let me get X-rays of your back and then call one of our orthopedic surgeons."

"No!" he shouted. He stood, bringing his six-foot-two-inch frame to full height. "Just the Demerol, Captain. Then I'll be gone."

"I'm afraid I can't do that, sir, not until I've completed your evaluation."

"Captain, this is the military. You do as I say. Understand?" His voice was now crisp and direct.

My pulse jumped. "Will twenty pills be enough to get you through this attack, sir?"

It was a slow day in surgery, so I was pulled for a shift in the outpatient clinic. The portly woman in her thirties, a lieutenant's wife, was my third patient. The crisis was her stuffy nose. "I want my cold-pack. And my son's getting a stuffy nose. Write him a prescription for one too. We're entitled."

If there was anything about the military that raised my blood pressure, it was the cold-pack: a combination of over-the-counter decongestant tablets, nose drops, throat lozenges, and a box of Army-issue facial tissues. All of it was available at any local pharmacy without a prescription. But that wasn't good enough. On base, the cold-pack was free. And because it was free, we had a constant stream of family members desperate for a cold-pack.

My father once said that if I wanted to see what socialized medicine would be just look at the military. I'd thought a lot about the differences between military and civilian medical care. To the military, health care services were a right. Outside the military, however, there just wasn't enough money to cover everyone. I was certain that giving out cold-packs at the first sign of a sniffle wasn't the answer.

A corpsman burst in to the exam area. "Captain, they need you over in the operating room. STAT!" I pushed the two prescriptions at the lieutenant's wife and rushed out.

After six months without anyone to help me with anesthesia, the Army transferred in a nurse anesthetist to fill John's position until he returned from his surgery leave. Major Len Reeves's arrival was a gift. The Major became a close friend. He was also a great technician, with eighteen years' experience. We learned from each other. Len appreciated my understanding of pathophysiology, while I benefited from his years of experience.

I ran down the long wooden hall connecting the several World War II Army barracks that had been tied together to create Fort Benjamin Harrison's hospital. I could think of the often-quoted adage: *Anesthesia is hours of boredom mixed with moments of stark terror.* I rushed through the swinging doors into the sterile area.

"What happened?" I called out to Len.

"I can't ventilate him. He was doing fine, and then I couldn't get any air through."

I looked over at the surgeon, an ENT (ear, nose, and throat) specialist. He said, "It's just a routine partial thyroidectomy in an otherwise healthy forty-year-old male. No extra bleeding."

"Did you give him more sucs?" I asked Len. Sucs was a paralyzing drug, succinyl choline, routinely used to keep patients immobile during surgery. My mind raced to find a solution. This was the moment I'd feared since arriving at the post. Other than the possibility of bronchospasm, which should have been relieved by an extra bolus of the paralyzing agent, I drew a blank.

I grabbed the rubber ventilating bag and squeezed. Nothing! Afraid to remove the endotracheal tube and lose our only possible airway, I called out to the ENT doctor. "Trach him!"

The procedure took another two minutes until I could pull out the old tube and slip a new one into the exposed tracheotomy site. We were now able to ventilate the patient, but despite external cardiac massage and added oxygen, we were unable to revive him. After ten minutes, I called off our resuscitative effort. We were too late. I pulled the sheet over his face. I was devastated. So was everyone else in the operating room. Not because we hadn't done our best, but because our best wasn't good enough.

I picked up the old endotracheal tube, hoping for an answer. Immediately, I recognized a problem. The balloon that was supposed to prevent leakage of oxygen from around the rubber tube had slipped down to the end, blocking off the opening. I felt sickened. In my brief training and the almost eight months I had been at the hospital, I had never seen or heard of that happening. Whether that was the cause of the patient's demise or it had occurred while I was pulling out the tube, I'd never know.

Lt. Col. Peaves said, "The soldier has a wife and two young kids out in the waiting room. Which one of you is going to tell them?"

Without a word, we all headed for the swinging doors to the waiting room area. Despite the tragic outcome, we were a team.

Life at the hospital marched on, but it was my life at home that kept me on edge.

Janet had finally conceived. Early in her pregnancy, she had been besieged by nausea, but with Bendectine for her and an almost constant diet of Big Macs for me, we made it through. At six months, Janet started spotting and had to be hospitalized. Fortunately, the bleeding did not turn out to be the dreaded placenta previa, which would have required a cesarean section. We discovered that her placenta was situated near the edge, instead of over the opening of the cervix. Captain Alex Rodriguez, her obstetrician, called it a marginal placenta. He felt she could go to term if she took it easy. Two weeks later, she experienced more bleeding, but it stopped on its own after some much needed bed rest. Planning for the upcoming delivery, we sent Trey back to Texas to stay with Janet's parents until our situation was more stable.

On a Monday, during the evening news, Janet said, "You better get a tub, or I'm going to leak all over the place." She said it as matter-of-factly as my father might have, and it reminded me of him. "My water just broke."

The day of reckoning was upon us. Although I never shared my concerns with Janet, I was unable to dispel the fear that once she started to dilate, the bleeding might become a problem. Just in case, I kept a large needle and a bottle of IV fluid in my briefcase.

When Janet's call went out, all my plans about transporting her to the hospital evaporated. She kept her composure, directing me to load the car while she stood dripping into the small plastic washtub.

As we pulled up to the emergency room doors, Janet said, "You ran one red light and two yellows getting us here. If I wasn't already in labor, after that ride, I am now."

"I'm going to ask Len to come in," I said. I turned Janet over to the nurse at the emergency entrance. We didn't routinely have anesthesia coverage for deliveries unless there was an expected problem. I disappeared in the direction of the operating room suite to change into scrubs.

I was on anesthesia call, but Len would come in for Janet's delivery. Both my calls to him went unanswered. I changed into scrubs and quickly made my way over to labor and delivery. According to the nurse, tonight was quiet, with one other mother in labor.

I entered Janet's small room.

"I'm having strong contractions," Janet said.

"Any bleeding?"

She shook her head. "The last contraction was two minutes ago. Another is starting."

I sat down in the chair beside her. "I couldn't locate Len. It looks like we'll be here for a while. I'll call him again later." I gazed at the wooden walls. "This setup doesn't give us much privacy, but the nurse said they only had one other woman in labor."

As I checked the 14-gauge Angiocath I'd requested, Alex sauntered through the door.

"I guess we're going to be in for a long night," he said. "Maybe I can give you something to speed you up a little." He raised the sheet and slipped his hand beneath.

I settled back in the chair and opened the evening paper. I planned to give it another hour, and then call Len again.

"Alex, the paper says President Nixon may have our troops out of Vietnam within a year. You know what that means? We might not have to go."

"We have a problem." Alex quickly withdrew his bloodied hand from under the sheets. "You're dilated to eight centimeters. We have to move to delivery now!"

"We need Len," I said, but it was too late.

Alex grabbed the foot of Janet's bed and started pulling it through the door.

Janet was scuttled to delivery and shunted onto the table. Alex donned his gown and gloves and hurried to the foot of the table.

"Push," he said. "Push. Push."

I recalled the dictum about not being a doctor to one's own family, how a physician could lose objectivity when things went bad. I checked Janet's IV, turning up the drip slightly. I wrapped the blood pressure cuff around her arm and pumped. One twenty-six over eighty-two: a strong pulse. Everything was going well.

"Here, breathe this oxygen," I told her. "You're doing fine."

"One final push," Alex said.

The color in Janet's face vanished. "I'm going to faint," she said. Then she dropped off, no longer responsive.

I pumped the blood pressure cuff. The first beat I heard came in somewhere around sixty. I felt for a pulse over her carotid artery, thready but still palpable. I opened her IV to full and raised the IV pole as high as I could. I increased the flow of oxygen and began to ventilate her. At some point, I stopped thinking. I stopped listening. My movements were habit, adjusting this, twisting that. Time passed in a slow haze.

Alex's remark brought me back to reality. "Looks like all the parts are here." He held our baby up.

"Let me see." Janet's muffled voice was barely audible under the mask. "Is it a boy or a girl?" The color in her cheeks had returned.

I said, "A beautiful little girl."

15

FIFTEEN MINUTES EVERY TWO HOURS

———— ▪ ————

Resident Nixon withdrew our troops more rapidly than anyone anticipated. As a result, my orders to serve in Vietnam never came through, and I completed my tour of duty at Fort Benjamin Harrison. Although I never tasted the fear of combat, I left the Army a changed person. No longer would I automatically rely on someone else in case I got in trouble. No longer would I take for granted the sacrifices of our fighting forces. And never again would I write another prescription for a cold-pack.

My time in the Army gave me time to reflect on my career in medicine. With anesthesia, I was exposed to all types of surgery and quickly realized I was not cut out to be a plastic surgeon, or at least, not one who made his living doing cosmetic surgery. I didn't particularly enjoy the temperament of that type of patient. After ruminating over what I'd make out of my practice and my life, I settled on ophthalmology. Returning to my alma mater, I completed a three-year residency at Dallas' Parkland Hospital. I then joined a group of two other doctors who were opening an office in a new hospital in North Dallas. Janet, deep into raising Trey and our new daughter, Robyn, happily agreed with my decision, since we were close to home but not too close.

It had been two years since completing my residency, and my practice was starting to do well. My father's health was not.

He had recently retired, and at least a part of his planning had worked out well. His primary concern was leaving his patients in good hands. Fortunately, he had received an offer from a young Dallas surgeon who had become disenchanted with the trappings of a big city practice. It was a perfect fit, since the doctor had come from a small town in the Midwest. The money from the sale of his practice was enough to pay off the loan on the small building where his office was located across the street from the hospital. The little left over, he stashed in his savings account. As far as my father was concerned, he received more than a suitable return. He considered the practice a gift from my grandfather and the other doctors who had referred him their patients.

With each visit, my father's deteriorating health became more obvious. Although my mother now openly discussed his difficulty breathing, the cause of his condition was never a topic of conversation. The whole family was in denial, faulting bad genes, since my father's mother died of emphysema and claimed she never smoked a day in her life. Even at this stage, it appeared that my father seemed more concerned that my mother didn't discover he had lied about giving up smoking.

I'd pulled an all-nighter suturing up a lacerated eye from a bar fight when my mother telephoned. She and my father had cut short their trip to Padre Island. The getaway was meant to celebrate his retirement and was intended to be a fresh start, symbolic of a new life, free from the obligations of more than forty uninterrupted years dedicated to medicine.

I said, "I didn't think you were due back until next week."

"Your father caught a cold last week," she said. "He just couldn't shake it. We saw this doctor who felt he might be getting pneumonia. He wanted to put him in the hospital down there." She let out a slow deep breath. "You know your father. He felt if anyone was going to take care of him, it was going to be Dr. Hearn. So, here we are. We're supposed to be at his office at ten tomorrow morning."

Morton Hearn, an internist who was part of a group that practiced at Baylor Hospital, had been my father's doctor for as long as I could remember. I never understood their connection, but from my father's point of view, the relationship worked well. My father would describe to Hearn what he felt was wrong with him, usually over the telephone, and Hearn, most of the time, would answer him with what he wanted to hear. It was like volleying a tennis ball against a brick wall—the return totally dependent on what you put into the shot. Hearn was a good enough guy, well respected in the local medical circles.

"Maybe he needs a good shot of penicillin," I said, trying to mask my growing concern.

"I'll call you after he sees Dr. Hearn."

At that moment I picked up on the shifting roles of their relationship. Although he had relied on my mother for support, my father had always been the dominant figure in the family. My mother followed close behind, dutifully smoothing out the ruts he left in his path. But all that was about to change.

I'll never forget the shock of seeing my father in the hospital. He was gaunt, pale, and weak. He sat on the side of the bed, his bare feet hanging nearly to the floor as he gasped for every bit of air his failing lungs could suck in.

I said, "I see they decided to keep you."

"Hearn put me on antibiotics," he puffed out, looking over at the IV bottle above his bed. "The problem is, I've had to be catheterized, and it's killing me." His face contorted in pain as he reached up to adjust the oxygen mask that clung loosely across his face.

My father had undergone surgery to correct a prostate problem almost ten years before. I knew the medicines he was being given to help his breathing would cause urinary retention due to a relapse in his prostate condition. "That's just temporary until they can get your infection under control."

My mother was huddled in the far corner with a dingy, hospital blanket draped around her shoulders. The look on her face told me everything I needed to know about the state of my father's health.

"I've got to get it out *now!*" he almost screamed. "The damned thing is killing me!"

"We've put in a call to Dr. Hearn," my mother said, "to see if they can give him anything. The catheter has him so stirred up he can't think of anything else."

"You've got to be careful with pain medicines," I said to her, recalling how they dulled the respiratory centers in the brain. "If they give him too much it could shut down his . . ."

The door to my father's hospital room creaked open, and Morton Hearn stepped through. "Mayo, the nurses tell me you and that catheter aren't getting along."

"It's killing me."

"They had to put one in me about a year ago when I had my prostate reamed out. The first twenty-four hours were pretty rough." Hearn looked around at my mother and me. "Robbie, I hear good things about you out there at . . ."

"Medical City. Thanks, but you probably heard that from my parents."

"Never get out that far. Lots of new young doctors, I hear."

My office at Medical City Hospital was five miles up the highway from downtown Dallas. The dynamics of the city were changing, and a growing number in the community were looking north for their shopping and health care needs. Our hospital and office complex was born when a large group of physicians decided to close their downtown facility and move north. I was one of about fifty other young physicians, all hooked on to the established group's coattails, looking for a place to light. The medical complex resembled a hotel more than a hospital, and its style attracted younger people moving into North Dallas. The approach worked. Nonetheless, there were pockets of resentment from some of the older physicians. I couldn't tell where Dr. Hearn stood.

"If you ever want to visit," I said, "I'll be glad to show you around."

He ignored my offer. "Mayo, I'm going to give you something for pain so you can get some rest." It was then I first saw the syringe full of clear liquid clasped in his hand. He moved up to the head of the bed and quickly began to empty its contents into the IV tubing.

"Wait." I raised my hand. "With his emphysema, isn't that going to slow down his respiration?"

Hearn looked over at me. "As I recall, you're an ophthalmologist. You stick to eyes and let me worry about your father."

Within moments, my father slowly sank back onto his bed. Confused about whether I should be embarrassed or angry, I did nothing.

"Why don't we let Mayo get some rest," Dr. Hearn said. "You two might want to grab a bite in the cafeteria."

Baylor Hospital's cafeteria resembled most others—drab, carpetless, and unfriendly. The place reminded me of the school cafeterias of my earlier years in Waxahachie.

I thought I heard my family's surname over the hospital's intercom. Fifteen seconds later, there was no mistaking the operator's urgent message as she repeated it a second time. We were to report back to the floor where my father was located.

My mother dropped her nibbled toast, and we hurried to the elevators. As we exited the elevator, a nurse moved quickly toward us. "Dr. Hearn asked me to have you wait for him in the waiting room."

"What's wrong?" my mother asked.

The nurse stepped aside as a technician pushing a portable breathing machine rushed past her and into my father's room. "The doctors are with your husband now. As soon as they know something, they'll come out and talk to you."

"Doctors?" I said, relieved that Hearn was no longer acting alone.

"Dr. Garratt, one of our pulmonary specialists, and his resident are in there with Dr. Hearn. Now if you would please wait down there." She pointed to the end of the hall. "One of the doctors will see you shortly."

I gently tugged on my mother's arm. "They'll come get us," I said. "Hearn probably asked the pulmonologist in to see if there's anything else he should do. You know how Pop hates to be here. So, they're trying to get it all in before he decides to check himself out."

"I don't think so," she said. We slowly moved back toward the waiting area.

We'd barely settled in when a tall blonde man came toward us. "You must be Barbara. And you must be Mayo's son, the eye doctor. I'm Bill Garratt."

"What about my husband?"

"I'm afraid, not very good news." His look was solemn. Morton Hearn came up behind him. "We're moving him into the ICU," Garratt

121

said. We all turned as an orderly appeared down the hall dragging my father in his bed behind him. At the other end, with one hand on the bed and the other on the portable ventilating machine we had seen just moments before, was a young man in a white coat similar to Garratt's. "That's my resident. He'll stay with Mayo until we get him settled in the unit."

"We just left him thirty minutes ago," I said.

"He had a respiratory arrest."

"You mean he quit breathing, because his respirations were suppressed?"

"That's usually the way it happens," Garratt said. "The respiratory center in the brain can become so used to the oxygen deprivation that the slightest thing can turn it off."

Garratt sounded like one of my medical school professors. The situation reminded me of something my father used to say: "The most dangerous doctor is the one who doesn't know his own limitations." Too bad Morton Hearn hadn't listened to this bit of wisdom a little earlier.

"Such as with a dose of narcotic?" I looked over Garratt's shoulder at Morton Hearn, whose eyes were glued to the floor. Neither physician responded to my question. I hadn't expected they would.

It had been just over a week since father was admitted, and his condition was still touch and go. When I wasn't at work, I was at the hospital in the waiting area with my mother. Janet, at home with the kids, checked in regularly and even brought us dinner on several occasions. But with my father's health and my continuing responsibilities at work, I was drained of everything, including my appetite.

My sister, Susie, who was now a mother of her own with two boys, Rich and Ben, had been given many of the day-to-day decisions that concerned my parents' life back in Waxahachie. She had mentioned looking for a house in Dallas for them, an idea that was unthinkable just days before. My mother and I kept up the vigil at night and most evenings until after the last visitation period ended at ten o'clock. My father was so sick that I was not sure he knew we were there. But if only for our benefit, one of the family members made the trek into his cubicle each time the doors to the ICU opened, a visit that lasted exactly fifteen minutes on even-numbered hours.

We were not alone; family members of other patients in the ICU waited with us. Most of the time, we only talked about the weather or the temperature in the waiting area, a subject that had oddly taken on a great significance. Occasionally, we did share meaningful dialogue with these strangers, but it was usually brief and probably more a transference of our own uncertainties than true empathy for their loved ones.

On day five, the wife of a patient in the cubicle next to my father found out I was a doctor. As soon as we returned to the waiting area, she pumped me for everything I knew about her husband's condition. I tried to be optimistic. The next day his bed was filled with another very sick person. I learned he'd thrown a clot to his lung and been transferred to another part of the hospital.

At night, the large waiting room looked like an encampment. Blankets were the uniforms of choice as concerned family members and loved ones huddled together in small groups. No longer did our family think in terms of days, nights, or even weekends, but two-hour segments with the ten p.m. to eight a.m. hiatus the only break. As we communicated among ourselves, the consuming topic was my father's roller-coaster condition: his temperature, last oxygen level, even his urine output had become top priority. We would discuss and dissect every morsel of information we either gleaned from those brief visits or had tossed in our direction by his doctors and nurses. We relayed his vitals to other family members who were not at the hospital. It was as if we were acting as his surrogate doctors, using our wills and prayers to help heal him, one encouraging word or laboratory test at a time.

"Did Garratt come out yet?" my mother asked, a shadow of her former self, she fell into the sofa.

"He went in about thirty minutes ago," I said. "He'll check back with us before he goes home."

"He's always here," she said. "I don't know when he finds time for his family."

Just then, Dr. Garratt broke though the doors of ICU and headed in our direction. We stood up, clinging to each other.

"I think Mayo's going to make it," he said. "But the worst is not over." He looked away for a moment. "His condition is called Burger's disease. It's when the vessels to the legs shut down if the blood is needed by some other parts of the body. When Mayo was sick, what little blood his heart could pump went to protect his brain and the other vital organs."

"What are you trying to tell us?" my mother asked.

"He has gangrene of his feet. We tried everything we could." He stopped, slowly shaking his head.

"So what does that mean?" I was growing more frustrated by the endless crises.

"If we don't amputate your father's feet, he's going to die."

The surgery to remove both of my father's legs just below the knees went well, and by the day after surgery, with the toxins from the gangrenous tissue no longer poisoning his body, his vital signs were greatly improved. Although it was an emotional blow for the family, our overriding consolation was that we still had the part of him that mattered.

"You're beginning to look like your old self," I told him.

Still groggy from the anesthesia, he looked over, and gave me a weak grin, a positive sign. It was the first smile I could recall since he had entered the hospital. "Well, almost." His smile quickly faded as he looked down at the flattened sheets below his knees.

Throughout my life, I had been exposed to many people labeled disabled, but my father was the first who was close to me. To my embarrassment, up to now I had always thought of them as different, more deserving of my pity. Facing the uncertainties of my father's future, I realized there are two different situations that individuals with limiting conditions fall into: those made even stronger by the burden, and those who become truly disabled by it. Frequently, the only difference is their state of mind.

"Garratt tells me they're going to start physical therapy next week. Maybe even fit you with artificial legs the week after."

"I don't know if I can ever walk again. I don't know if I'm up to it. With my breathing the way it is and with my feet gone, I'm tired."

"You sound like some of your patients." I pulled up a chair and sat beside his bed. "When I first started following you around making rounds, I was no taller than this." I held my hand out level with his bed. "I didn't know anything about medicine except what I learned from you. I can still remember those patients moaning and complaining about their problems, but you didn't give them any choice. They were going to get well." I sat back. "Maybe, it's time you took your own advice."

16

STANDING AGAIN

————— ∎ ∎ —————

Two long months earlier, my mother had loaded my father into the car and brought him to Dallas. Now he was going home— not to their house of over twenty-five years; not even to another house in Waxahachie, the town where my father was born and spent all his life. They were going to a new home in Dallas, one close to my sister and me. Making the decision to move had been difficult for my mother. With my father's doctors located in Dallas, and with him now a bilateral amputee, my mother and father would need help. Difficult as it was to leave a place with a lifetime of memories, the move was their only logical choice.

"I see their car coming down the block!" my nephew, Rich, cried out, peering between the curtains of the living room window.

Janet and Susie, back in the kitchen, scurried to ready the chocolate cake, my father's favorite. After the endless days and nights of uncertainty, everyone was ready to celebrate the first day of my parents' new life.

The process of moving into their new home had turned into a family project. My sister found the house. Janet transformed the interior into their home. The rest of us joined in spending the better part of two weeks, working nights and weekends, cleaning, painting, and arranging wheelchair access before it was completed. Even the grandkids, our two and Susie's two, did their part. It was our gift to my parents in return for a lifetime of love and nurturing.

Rich ran to the front door. "They're here!"

My parents' car pulled up to the curb. I was somewhat nervous, but excited at the same time as we all poured out onto the porch. We'd had carpenters build a wheelchair ramp out the backdoor to the garage, but today was special. I was determined that my father was going to enter his new home for the first time through the front door, even if we had to carry him.

And that's what we had to do. After some tricky maneuvering to get him out of the car and into his new wheelchair, my brother-in-law, Pete, and I lifted him and his wheelchair up the concrete steps to the porch.

"You look almost as bad as I do," my father said, noticing how out of breath I was from the effort.

I grinned back at him. Suddenly his mask of self-control fell and tears rushed to his eyes. Fighting to hold back my own emotions, I eased in among the other members of the family as we watched him take in his new surroundings.

"I'll never be able to tell you what this means to me," he said. He made no attempt to wipe away the tears. "To be given a second chance, and now this."

"Do you want to go on in and see if we put everything where you want it?" I asked.

He nodded, unable to bring himself to speak. The grandkids rushed back through the door, toward the kitchen and the cake and ice cream, and the rest of the family quickly followed. I fell in behind his wheelchair and was beginning to push him forward when he held up his hand.

He looked up at me. "For whatever reason, I've been given this chance. I will walk again."

___ ▄ ▪ ▄ ___

Two weeks after the welcome home party, I received a call from my father. "I need for you to come over. The sooner the better."

Janet's growing frustration was painted across her face as she looked across the kitchen at me. In the background, I could see the kids clamoring at the table waiting for their dinner.

"I just walked in," I said. Even though Medical City was my main office, the group I'd joined had several other locations. As a doctor still developing his own practice, and with large gaps present in my schedule early on, it was the consensus that I try to pick up extra patients by taking on some of my partners' overflow at the other two offices. The plan was working, but it did make for some grueling days. "Let me grab something to eat and then I'll be right over."

"I want you to get rid of them."

"Get rid of what," I asked.

"You'll see when you get here."

By the time I arrived, a full hour had passed. "Janet needed help getting the kids to bed," I explained.

He was propped up in his wheelchair in the middle of a back bedroom that had been converted into his office.

"Just take them." He lifted a small wooden box he'd been cradling in his lap. "I don't want to see them again."

"What's in the box?"

"My amputation knives. I got them during the war. I never thought anyone would have to use knives like these on me." He looked down at the tightly wrapped stubs of his legs.

During World War II, my father had been assigned to a large evacuation hospital in France. Like many of the veterans who survived, he never talked about his experiences. I'd always assumed they were too painful. I took the wooden box from his outstretched hands.

"I guess I should say thank you," I said.

"I can't begin to count the number of times I used those during the war. Even used them here for a couple of years when I first got back, until the hospital bought me some newer ones." He looked away, a slight catch in his breathing. "I was trained to do amputations. Just cut off the patients' mangled limbs or what was left of them, making sure they didn't hemorrhage to death. Then pray they didn't die from gangrene. As far as I was concerned, if I'd done my job right, their problems were over. For most of them, the war was over. They were evacuated back to the States for rehabilitation before they were discharged."

"It's the way war works," I said. "You patch up the ones you can and send them on."

"That's what we're taught. But somewhere along the way, I think we missed something."

Several weeks later, I watched as he struggled through physical therapy. Sweat glistened off his deeply furrowed face as he pulled himself out of his wheelchair to a position between two elevated parallel bars. He stood perched atop his two artificial legs, beaming from ear to ear. "There!" he said.

When he first began physical therapy, his arms were so weak from his prolonged illness that they were almost no use. He was determined not to squander his second chance. It helped that Lindy, his therapist, was so encouraging. Having agreed to fill in on the Saturday shift while my mother took a well-deserved break, I watched from across the large room. Lindy cajoled him to take his first step away from the wheelchair.

"You can do it," Lindy said, sounding more like a cheerleader than a therapist. She had become the constant topic of conversation: what she said, what she wore, how her two children were doing in school. My parents' fixation wasn't so much with Lindy as with her link to my father's normalcy. She represented his conduit to a productive life.

"All you've got to do is put one foot in front of the other," I said from a distance.

"You try doing this on a pair of stilts and see how easy it is." Then he looked back at Lindy, who was holding out her arms just beyond his reach. "It hurts so bad to put weight on them."

"Dr. Mayo," Lindy said, "remember what Dr. Garratt told you. The only way you're going to get through that is to stand on them."

Lindy was referring to my father's stumps. Although his breathing difficulties were still of great concern, there was nothing more to do but maintain the status quo. So in the family's search for hope, our focus shifted to something we could affect: standing, walking. The health of his legs was his connection to a fuller life. We routinely agonized over the condition of the skin around his stumps, whether to use an ace wrap or cling gauze or both, the thickness of the special socks that went over the wrappings. These questions consumed us. The whole family was going through this recovery together. It was something that, as a doctor, I had never before realized.

Suddenly, one of my father's artificial legs swung forward. He let out a rush of air and brought the other up alongside. "Is that what you wanted me to do?"

"That's a good start. Now you need to do something else for me." Lindy's bright eyes darted to the bottom of his prostheses, which were fitted in a pair of his old loafers.

"What?" My father's arms were tightly wrapped around the parallel bars.

"Since it looks like you're going to be doing a great deal of walking around here, you need to buy you some new shoes."

■

Since my father's release from the hospital, every call from my parents sent my stomach into knots. Our family's unpredictable situation had opened up a whole new perspective for me. I now knew what it was like on the receiving side of medicine, and it was a lot scarier than I'd imagined. Wondering whether my father's next cold would be his last, waiting for the next visit to the doctor, and fearing what we'd find out.

There were days when the pressure got to me. Fortunately, Janet's presence gave me stability.

One day, I received a call from my mother. "I think your father needs some help."

When I arrived, I asked. "What's going on?"

"We went shopping today for your father's new shoes." My mother was ladling broth over a chicken she was roasting in the oven. "They're really fancy for your father, tassels and everything. I think Lindy is going to love them."

"So what's the problem?"

"He won't let me help him." She turned back to the stove. "Said he has to do it himself. I thought maybe you could change his mind."

I headed toward the back room where my father spent virtually all his waking hours. As I approached, a faint smell of perfume began to tickle at my nose.

I poked my head through the door. "What's up?"

"It's Johnson's," he answered without looking up. "Baby powder."

My father was coated with a thick layer of white dust. Moving closer, I could see his prosthesis positioned under his arm. A dusty black sock covered the artificial foot. In his right hand, he gripped one of his new shoes.

"The guy that sold them said there'd be no problem getting them on." He dumped another shake of powder into the shoe then crammed the foot of the prosthesis into it. After a brief struggle, the slippery shoe fell to the floor. My father looked down helplessly.

"Want some help?"

He handed me his artificial leg. I plopped down on the sofa and began to go through the same exercise with similar results. "I think the salesman sold you the wrong size shoes." Sweat began to rim my brow. "Why didn't you just let him put them on for you then?"

"He did, but I had on the wrong socks."

My mother appeared at the door. "Want some motherly advice?"

"I don't think they fit," I said.

She held up a shiny object. "You might want to try this. They say it works wonders."

"What's that?" I asked.

"I believe they call it a shoehorn."

———— ∎ ————

In the months that followed, we had gotten back in the habit of weekly Sunday get-togethers. Janet and Susie had offered their homes for the dinners, but since our houses weren't set up for wheelchair access, it was easier for all of us to come to our parents'.

Entering the house, I balanced the squash casserole in one hand while holding the door for Janet and the kids with the other.

"Susie and the family should be on their way over," my mother said, taking the dish as the kids scrambled by her. "Your father has a new job at the hospital. He's been asked to speak to the other physical therapy patients about overcoming their difficulties."

"Where is he?"

"In the kitchen."

I found my father staring out the kitchen window.

"I heard about the job," I said.

He beamed proudly. "I guess they think I can make a difference."

"The old professor in you coming out," I said.

My father was a natural teacher and loved being in front of an audience. It was his love, but in some ways, also the source of his greatest frustration because he couldn't afford to do it full time—not and uphold his responsibilities to us, his family, and his father. He frequently reminded me he would have been an actor if it had not been for his father prodding him to go into medicine.

After graduating from Harvard Medical School, my father had aspirations of going into academia, where he could teach, but World War II brought those plans to a halt. Grossly overworked, my grandfather coaxed him back to Waxahachie after the war, telling him that his stay there would be temporary and another doctor would eventually take his place. Years and thousands of operations later, that replacement had yet to come. With his family entrenched in their own lives, it was too late to make a mid-career change. This new opportunity might not only propel him along his path of recovery, but also get him back to his first love.

A camera hung from his neck. Prior to his illness, it had been a constant companion at family events.

"I see you dusted off your camera," I said.

"Thought I might take some pictures of the grandkids," he said. He picked up the camera and aimed it at me. "They may gripe now, but someday they're going to appreciate them."

"Want me to roll you in there?" I asked.

Suddenly his expression changed. "I'll do it!" He dropped the camera onto his lap, grabbed the wheels and spun around toward the den.

"I was trying to help."

"You need to give me the opportunity to do what I can for myself."

Then I realized that maybe the most important part of my father's recovery was not getting his strength back or learning how to walk again, but his ability to regain his self worth. By treating him as a burden, I was delaying his recovery.

He moved the wheelchair forward, but stopped to glance back

over his shoulder. "It looks like the ladies have everything under control. Why don't you make yourself useful and help me take these pictures?"

(17)

A Lifetime Commitment

M y parents' car was retrofitted with hand controls for the foot pedals so my father could drive. The car and all the new gadgets had arrived back from the dealership only yesterday. The whole family was planning to gather on Sunday to celebrate the event as one more step in my father's road to recovery. Unfortunately, he'd crashed the car into the garage door earlier in the day.

"He didn't make it out of the driveway," my mother said. "Personally, I think it's kind of funny, going forward when he should have gone backward. But your father doesn't look at it that way. He sees it as a failure."

"What do you want me to do?" I asked.

She laid the last dinner plate back on the shelf and closed the cabinet door. "Just try to cheer him up. Tell him it's no big deal. The people from Sears are coming out tomorrow to replace the door, and I talked to Lynn Langley down at the insurance company. He tells me they'll cover everything but the deductible."

"With what he's just been through, this shouldn't bother him that much."

"He's not used to being dependent on others."

My mother wasn't the only sad one. We were all having difficulty with his amputations. How he looked when he stood up. How many steps, balanced upon his mechanical legs, he could take on his own.

135

How he got in and out of bed. Even how he got on and off the commode. As a family, we had become consumed with the idea of helping him get back to normal.

"I'll see what I can do." I headed off down the hall. The muted sounds of the television grew louder as I approached the back room. "Mother tells me you had a run-in with the garage door today."

"It seems I pulled when I should have pushed. That's what happens when you give a surgeon a choice."

"How's that?"

"Internists, well, they can spend all day agonizing over a decision—do I order this test or that? Do I start this medicine or that? Surgeons are wired differently. When we're presented with a problem, we don't waste time stewing over what we're going to do. By the time they decide, it could be too late."

"But you took out the garage door because you hadn't learned the controls."

"An internist wouldn't have even tried to get behind the wheel."

I smiled. Despite his apparent setback, the gaping hole in the garage door was testimony that my father was getting back to normal.

"Since you're here, I want to show you something." My father rolled over to his desk and pulled open the bottom drawer on the right side. "This is where I've stored my important papers—the ones I want to keep private."

"Shouldn't all those papers be put in the safety deposit box?"

"How would I get them if I needed them? I can't just hop in the car and run down to the bank. I've categorized them according to their level of importance."

The tabs on the file folders had different colored writing. "I see you're back to using your colored fountain pens." I was referring to the letters he sent me in college with words and sentences underlined in different colors to emphasize the points he wanted to make.

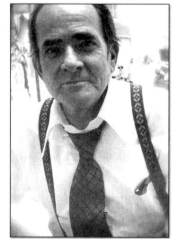
Dr. Mayo

"It helps me locate what I need in a hurry. These here are *Private*. Those are our insurance policies and documents relating to the ownership of the house and car. Next, the *Very Private* papers are in green, such as our stock certificates and bank balances."

I read the yellow letters on the next tab. "What are your *Extremely Private* papers?"

He straightened in his wheelchair, but did not look up. "Those are wills and contracts with the funeral home about our burial plots."

He had come so close to cashing in on that contract just months ago. His brush with death and the continuing deterioration of his pulmonary status was a subject we had only touched on since he had been released from the hospital. "And what about that final category?"

"*Most Private*," he read out loud. "That's my curriculum vitae. It has all the important information on me from college to medical school. I even included my teaching in the rehabilitation department over at the hospital. I've included the picture of me when I was president of the Texas Medical Association." He pushed the drawer closed and slowly rolled away from his desk. "I can't ask your mother to handle everything at that time. It's important to me that the newspaper gets it right. I'm going to rely on you and your sister for that."

My father called me at home. "You got a minute?"

"Sure." I flopped down on the bed. Voices of Janet and the kids echoed somewhere off in the house.

"Ben and Libby Carpenter were by here to check on me earlier today. They said your waiting room was almost full when they came in to have their eye exams."

I remembered that my parents' best friends had arrived in my office at a time when I was tied up with an emergency. They waited almost an hour to be seen for their scheduled appointment. "They complained they had to wait, didn't they?"

"On the contrary, they were impressed there were so many other patients who wanted to see you."

"How ironic. People want to see me *because* I'm busy."

I realized the same dynamics applied to the professional world.

When I first opened my office, patients saw me only because they couldn't get in to their own doctor. Often my waiting room stood empty. More than a few asked if they should get a second opinion. Some sought one. I wrote it off to my youthful appearance and my lack of experience. Now, only two years later, the patients were much more trusting of my treatment suggestions, often passing on accolades about my being up on the latest advances because I was fresh out of training. Just as I struggled to maintain my confidence in those early days, now I struggled to contain my over-confidence.

"Doctors have an obligation to try to keep on schedule," my father said, "but, by its very nature, the practice of medicine makes that difficult. It's an unpredictable science. Emergencies set us behind, and certain patients just need more time than we predicted. The rule I try to follow is that once I'm in the room with a patient, he or she is the only one I'm concerned about. Even if that means I spend a few extra minutes addressing their concerns."

"Running late keeps me on edge," I said. "Is that all you wanted to talk about?"

"Not exactly. It's normal for doctors to pat themselves on the back when they finally reach that stage in their careers when they think they've made it. But we wouldn't have gotten to where we are without the help of a lot of people who went before us. Take the antibiotics you dispense or the last operation you performed. They didn't just appear out of nowhere."

"I'm not sure what you're trying to tell me."

"For generations, doctors and their patients have struggled so that you and I could have the benefit of those medical breakthroughs."

"I'm so busy some days that I barely have time to think."

"That's how we all feel," he said. "Your medical education, how do you think you got it?"

"I earned it!" I recalled the countless hours I spent in lectures and holed up with all my books and notes.

"Ever thought of volunteering?" he asked.

"Is that what this is about?"

My father often boasted that the volunteer doctors' organizations kept our government from socializing medicine. He felt doctors working together could convince lawmakers that more rules didn't amount to better health care.

"Being a physician is also about giving something back," he said. His tone softened. "Why don't you give it a try? Volunteer for a committee at the County Medical Society and see how it feels."

My father's message haunted me. He and my grandfather had influenced me in many ways. Clearly, I wanted to be like them. I just didn't want to be them. I had turned out to be the doctor my father wanted. But now a selfless volunteer; I had to give it more thought.

The following day, I pulled into the hospital parking lot at Medical City. Off in the distance, the sound of a siren made me wonder what broken soul lay strapped to a gurney. It was a scene I'd lived since my earliest memories. At the end of that ambulance ride, someone was always there to help.

One side of me agreed with my father: it might be the time for me to give something back. But another side of me resisted, a side that saw my classmates from college who had chosen other professions and now expected their rewards. Why was medicine any different?

I stepped out of my car and headed toward the back entrance to the hospital. I was scheduled to be in the office in fifteen minutes and still had three patients to discharge from yesterday's surgery. I sidestepped the ambulance that had just arrived and caught sight of the patient, her face covered by an oxygen mask.

I realized my father was right. Our health care system didn't happen on its own. Countless doctors and nurses made a commitment to serve their patients over personal reward. I was party to that commitment. Maybe I'd earned my way, or maybe my opportunity was a gift from those who were willing to share their knowledge and experience. In either case, if I was going to be the type of physician my father expected of me, I had a long way to go.

18

LETTING MY FATHER GO

O ver the next three months, the emphysema took its toll on my father. The changes were subtle—a sallow look in his cheeks, lapses in memory. He fought hard to put on a good show, but his decline was obvious.

My mother did her best. Out of concern for my father's precarious condition, any member of the family with a respiratory illness was banished from my parents' home. Our kids, and the school they attended, were a breeding ground for infectious diseases; my parents would often go for long stretches without seeing them. As extreme as it sounded, I was convinced my mother's sheltering was the reason my father was able to survive the eighteen months since leaving the hospital, months that were some of the most meaningful our family shared. From that brief time, we learned that relationships mattered more than things.

In late afternoon, my mother called. She was breathless and seemed confused. "Dr. Garratt wants to put your father in the hospital. He's been on antibiotics for two days, but his fever hasn't broken. Your father doesn't want to go, but I didn't give him any other choice. Garratt said it would be a couple of days to clean him up, and then he would send him back home."

"Clean him up" was a term used to describe the process of treating the upper passages of my father's lungs.

"I'll come over and drive the two of you to the hospital."

"No! We can make it."

I had watched my mother grow stronger as my father weakened. She had become the dominant figure in their relationship as my father now devoted his energy to tying up the loose ends in his life—the deed to their new home, his will, and my mother's health care coverage.

"Are you sure?" I asked.

"No! I mean it!" This time her tone was more emphatic. "I have to take him myself. We'll call when we know the room number." The line went dead.

I realized the significance of her response, and my eyes filled with tears.

By the time I met my mother and father at Baylor Hospital, they were already situated in his room.

In the hall, I ran into Dr. Garratt. We hadn't seen each other in more than two years.

"You're Mayo's boy aren't you?" Dr. Garratt asked.

"How is he?"

I'd forgotten how tall he was. Swathed in a full length lab coat, a starched collar, and a perfectly knotted tie, he gave off the aura of omniscience. "I'm afraid we're going to have to put in a catheter. The medicines we've given your father to improve his breathing have caused him to go into acute urinary retention."

"The last time the catheter bothered him so much, Hearn had to give him narcotics to settle him down, and that's when he went into respiratory arrest. I think you know the rest."

"I'm afraid we don't have much choice." His voice was a whisper. He signaled for me to follow him as he moved further down the hall to a small alcove. "Your father has had a couple of good years, but his health has worsened."

"I'd hoped there was another answer," I said.

"The resistance to the blood flow through Mayo's lungs from his emphysema has become so high that it has finally caused the right side of his heart to fail." Garratt made me feel like I was back in medical school only this time the subject of discussion was not some unnamed patient buried in a textbook. "We've started him on digitalis and diuretics to try to take the load off his heart, but right now his electrolytes are still off the chart. If we don't get the pressure off his bladder, the pain and his elevated potassium will kick him into an irreversible cardiac arrhythmia."

"Isn't there anything else you can do? The minute you put in the catheter, he's going to go crazy until he gets the narcotics, and then his breathing is in trouble."

Garratt shook his head. "We can probably hold off for an hour. Go down there and see him. He told me he wants to talk to you."

When he turned to leave, I briefly caught a moist look in his eyes. Garratt's parting glance provided me more hope than anything he'd told me. I knew he still cared.

——— ▪ ———

I opened the door into my father's room.

"Come on in," my mother said.

I squinted through the darkness. All I could see was the luminescent glow of the cardiac monitor above my father's bed. "How's he doing?"

"As well as can be expected," my father's gravelly voice cut in. "Your mother made me come."

My mother rose from her chair in the corner and wrapped her arms tightly around my waist. Her frail body trembled. "Your father has something he wants to say to you."

A chill coursed through me as she closed the door behind her. I watched as he reached for the hand rail, struggling to right himself on the side. "Except for my smoking habit, I've never lied to you. So I'm not going to start now."

I watched as he sucked at the oxygen mask strapped across his face. "I talked to Garratt."

He lifted a hand to cut me off. "Someone from urology is coming over in a couple of minutes to put in a catheter. You remember what happened the last time?"

I nodded knowing, with a year-and-a-half more for the emphysema to ravage his weakened body, the chances he would pull out of respiratory failure were guarded at best.

"There're some things I need to go over with you while I still can. Your mother has always been at my side when it came to making the important decisions. Sometimes I think I made them, and sometimes I think she just let me think I made them. Looking back, it really didn't matter. The first time I met your mother, I thought she was the most beautiful thing in the world. When she agreed to marry me and move to Texas, I promised I would never do anything to make her regret that decision. The way it's worked out, I feel I've broken that promise. Through my own weakness, I threw away some of the best years of our lives together."

I groped for a response and finally gave up. I watched as he fought for each breath.

"Now, I'm asking you to step in for me. She's going to want to make her own decisions. It's her way of coping with the fact that she'll be alone. All I want you to do is be there when she needs you."

I choked back my tears. "I will." I felt an unbearable weight on my shoulders. My father was my support system, too.

"Being a patient is the hardest thing I've ever done," he said. "Your grandfather wasn't very good at it either. Maybe it's because we both know that doctors can't always make everything right, but you've still got to trust them." He rolled toward me and reached for my hand. "Whether it's your family or your patients, never betray their trust."

I realized that in one breathless sentence, my father had shared with me the final pronouncement that would carry me through the rest of my life. Although my grief was choking me, I now felt a strange sense of peace from this last bit of fatherly advice.

Hoping to stretch these final minutes into hours, I clung to his hand. The door to my father's room slipped open as a technician poked his head through. "Sir, Dr. Garratt sent me over from urology to put in the catheter."

"Give me a few more minutes," my father said. "Would you go get your mother for me? I need to see her one more time."

I turned to go.

He said, "That information in my '*most private*' file. Make sure the newspapers get it right."

Each day thereafter the news was worse. Despite a vast array of medications and IV fluid adjustments, his electrolytes continued to spiral out of control because of his failing kidneys. His body was shutting down. It was now only a matter of time.

My mother was huddled in an overstuffed chair in the far corner of the waiting area. I searched for a place to sit nearby that wasn't taken or littered with belongings of other families. "Did you see Dr. Garratt?" I asked.

"I think he's avoiding me. He sent us a message through Silverman," a wet-behind-the-ears intern who had befriended my parents. "I wanted to wait in your father's room so I could talk to Garratt directly. But the nurses sent me away so they could give him a sponge bath."

"It's probably that he's so busy."

"Yesterday, I saw him down the hall. I tried to signal him, but he looked right through me. He waited to see your father until after I left for dinner." She drew in a deep breath and pulled her knees up under the blanket. "He might think I blame him."

"What did Dr. Silverman say?"

"She said Dr. Garratt was trying to decide whether or not to start dialysis. He's leaving that decision up to us," she said.

"Us! Hell, he's the doctor. Isn't he supposed to tell us what to do?" My mind was a blur of contradictions. I wanted my father to live, but the physician in me knew that dialysis would only delay the inevitable. My first priority was to ensure he did not suffer, and I wasn't sure I could find the courage to make that decision. I wanted Garratt to make it for us.

"If you ask me, Garratt is shirking his duties."

"Some people do better under difficult situations, and doctors are no exception." My mother always looked for the good in people, rationalizing away their weaknesses. "I want to get Garratt alone and tell him I understand how he feels. One thing I've learned from being a doctor's wife for almost forty years: patients don't always get well. And all that we can ever ask of him is that he do everything he can."

"So what do we tell Dr. Silverman?"

"Your father is very tired. He's spent the better part of his life thinking about what's best for us. Now it's time we let him rest." I sensed a serenity come over her as she faced the most difficult

145

decision of her life. "Don't you think he's earned it?"

Even without the dialysis, my father held on for several days. The person trapped inside that dying body didn't feel like my father anymore. Numbed by the narcotics that allowed him to tolerate the catheter, his body was with us, but not his soul. His essence had moved on. I never thought I'd feel the way I did, but when his death finally came it was a relief. As a doctor, I had been trained to preserve life. The ravages of my father's disease taught me that's not always best. Now I understood there was a time to let the ones we care for go.

My father's passing had changed the way I viewed my responsibilities as a physician. The vocation of a doctor was not primarily to save lives, but to minimize suffering. Our forefathers understood that premise better than doctors of today. Armed with only a smattering of palliative potions, these practitioners traveled where they were needed. Sometimes their expertise changed the outcome. Often all they had to offer was a caring hand to hold. But in all cases, I believe their presence made a difference.

My heroes, my grandfather and my father, were gone. Strangely, their influence on me is greater in death than in life. I often recall my father poised over the young girl run over by a boat motor as his hands deftly closed her wounds. I recall my grandfather standing in defiance of racial bigotry when he opened, then closed, the Annex. My grandfather and father were exceptional physicians in their day. To me, however, their true legacy lay in their dedication. They gave of themselves regardless of outcomes and rewards. The practice of medicine was their life.

PART THREE

ON MY OWN

19

GONE FOR THE DAY

———— ▪ ————

After two decades of practicing medicine, I discovered that much of my work was repetitive. The same diseases, the same treatments, the same explanations—all that changed were the patients. On many levels, I had to admit that the honeymoon of my practice was over. I recalled my father telling me that every job becomes repetitious. "But keep in mind," he said, "what is routine to you is a new and frightening situation to your patients." To counterbalance my daily duties, I had become involved in the Dallas County Medical Society and the Texas Medical Association.

With our kids off at college, Janet and I now spent a great deal of time commuting between their campuses and lugging their belongings back and forth for the summer recesses. We even bought a small place on a lake in East Texas where I could refuel on weekends.

Then each Monday I would return to the office. Julie Chapman was the last patient of the day. She had almost no vision in her right eye, and the outside half of her left was starting to fail. Her problem was serious. I worried about a brain tumor or even a stroke, but kept my conversation general. Without further testing, I could do nothing more. She sat on her hands and tried to put on a brave front. Only her eyes gave her away. Her three-year-old son played with a pad and crayons in the corner of the examining room, while her infant daughter cried for attention in the stroller.

Julie reached into her purse, pulled out a tissue, and wiped her infant's runny nose. "I'm so sorry. I couldn't find a sitter."

"That's not a problem. Your children are welcome here."

"How bad is it? My eyes, I mean."

"We'll have to wait until tomorrow. We'll talk after you see the specialist."

She wanted an answer now. I could only imagine her torment confronting her loss of sight while her children still needed her full attention.

"Let me make a call," I said. I hoped to catch Dr. Taylor, a neurologist on the floor below. Although I was not certain of her exact diagnosis, I knew it was not life threatening, and delaying her workup until in the morning wouldn't affect her outcome. Nonetheless, a curbside consult with the neurologist couldn't hurt. I left Julie and her children in the examining room and went to make the call.

I got Dr. Taylor's receptionist on the phone.

"I'm sorry," she said, her tone indifferent, "but Dr. Taylor has gone for the day."

"Do me a favor? This lady is really upset. All she needs is a little reassurance. Check in the back office and see if he's still there. If he is, just ask him to give me a call. I don't think he needs to see her today, just some advice to hold her over until tomorrow."

The line went dead.

Overhearing my conversation, one of our technicians said, "Dr. Taylor is still here. I just passed him in the hall, heading back toward his office. I heard him say something about catching up on paperwork."

I returned to Julie with the good news: Dr. Taylor was still in the office. He would contact me shortly. The minutes dragged on as we awaited Dr. Taylor's call. After half an hour, I placed another call to his office. This time I was patched through to his answering service.

"I'm sorry," the operator came back. "Dr. Taylor must be gone. Do you want me to contact the doctor who's covering his calls?"

When I told Julie we'd missed Dr. Taylor, her eyes glistened. I hadn't asked for much from Dr. Taylor, a few reassuring words I could pass along. It appeared that was more than he or his receptionist was willing to give. I thought back to Waxahachie and our family's missed vacation to the coast when my father was caring for a patient. He'd said we were never able to step out of the role of doctor after we took the Hippocratic Oath.

Julie rose from the chair and began to pack up her son's crayons and coloring book. "Mommy, can we go to McDonald's on the way home?"

"We'll see."

"Please."

"All right. If that makes you happy."

In the following days, we discovered that Julie had a pituitary tumor, and her treatment began. I was struck by the irony that unlike Dr. Taylor, the mother in Julie was never *gone for the day*.

■ ■ ■

Mrs. Peavy was a middle-aged woman with a chronic eyelid infection. She was confused and slow to understand my instructions. She sat in the examining chair as I explained our treatment plan.

"Mrs. Peavy, we'll try this antibiotic for two weeks," I said.

"And then?"

"I'll check your eyes and see if the antibiotic is working."

"If it's working? In what way?"

I fought to suppress a yawn, a gesture forbidden to physicians when communicating with a patient. "We'll see if it clears up your infection."

"My eyes, you mean?"

As we exited, my technician whispered under her breath, "You told her the same thing twice." Embarrassed, I hoped Mrs. Peavy hadn't noticed. Lately, I'd caught myself drifting.

"Doctor," Mrs. Peavy called from the hallway. "Do I use this three or four times a day?"

"Four," I said. My patience was thin. It had been a long day, and I still had a waiting room full of patients. My assistants had cajoled me to shorten my explanations, telling me to give the patients preprinted materials outlining their medical problems and proposed treatments. So far, I'd resisted. A couple more Mrs. Peavys, and I might reconsider my position.

The fact was that I was bored.

According to my father, it happened to everyone. Through the years, he'd seen doctor after doctor reach a point of frustration with their practices. Everyone did. He described it as a moment when you discovered you had everything you thought you always wanted, and you still weren't satisfied. The solution to late-career boredom, he told me, was to refocus on the journey. What mattered wasn't getting there; it was the challenge of the expedition.

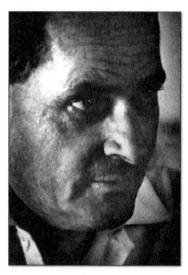

Dr. Mayo
Compliments of the Amon Carter Museum
Photographer: Nell Dorr

"If that doesn't help," he said, "then do what most doctors do and develop outside interests." I remember detecting a note of sadness in his voice.

He said, "When I first decided on medicine, I had dreams of helping people. During the rigors of medical school, some of those dreams got lost. During the war, I lost a few more. However, when I returned, I knew I had to make up to my family for all the years of sacrifice. I felt I owed a debt to them. Those early years weren't about recognition or money. They were about the journey. That's the trouble with many young doctors, they're trying to squeeze as many patients as possible into an already crowded schedule. They think a fancier car and jewelry for their wives will make them happy. It won't." My father had a way of pacing when he spoke. "Being a doctor has never been about the money or the prestige, or even the disease. It's about the patient."

I turned and strode down the hall where Mrs. Peavy was waiting to check out. "Would you like for me to go over those directions one more time?" I asked.

■ ■ ■

In the spirit of enjoying the journey, I took up tennis. All it got me was a gnawing bursitis in my shoulder. When the pain wouldn't go away, I sought professional help from an orthopedist named Clayton

Bennington. I was late for my appointment, and I tried to explain my tardiness to Dr. Bennington's receptionist, Marge.

"A patient wouldn't let me go," I said.

Marge wasn't buying it. She glared back at me as I grabbed for the pen on the sign-in sheet.

"That's why we schedule appointments, Doctor. I'm sure you expect the same from your patients. Now, if you would please have a seat, Dr. Bennington will get to you as soon as he can." She swiftly slid the glass partition shut.

I looked around for a seat in the crowded waiting room and saw one in the far corner. I slid into the chair next to a man in stained overalls.

"A real bitch, that one," he murmured. "She gave me the same song and dance when I got here. I told her my car broke down."

"Sometimes, we all have a bad day."

"Every day is a bad day for Marge. She was the same last week." He looked at the clock on the wall. "My appointment was over an hour and a half ago. Bennington is a nice enough guy, but he told me he'd given up trying to stay on schedule a long time ago. He said that with all the interruptions, it was impossible. If he wasn't the only doctor on my insurance plan, I wouldn't put up with this crap. Hell, my time is as valuable as his."

I'd heard similar complaints from my own patients. I wanted to tell him that the practice of medicine isn't an exact science; it's unpredictable, sometimes clumsy, and an often time-consuming art. That the best laid plans frequently go awry when determining how long a particular encounter will take. Maybe a patient has one extra question or a borderline test result that needs explaining. Then there are the emergencies, telephone calls from other physicians, hassles with insurance companies, plus the time I spent explaining to disgruntled patients why I made them wait. It all takes time.

I remember my father telling me that when a patient had an appointment with him, he took on a responsibility, not necessarily to see them at a designated time, but to allow enough time to ensure that their concerns were addressed before he moved on.

Some doctors, like Bennington, because of the apparent futility of trying to maintain a schedule, give up and become indifferent about their delays.

Then there was Marge, whose belligerent ways did little to allay the frustration of Bennington's patients. I knew another bulldog like her, also with a bun on her head, who ran the office for old Doc Hayes. Everyone in Waxahachie talked about how mean she was to Doc's patients. According to one story, if they smelled bad, she made the patients wait outside until the doctor was ready, even if they had a fever and it was the dead of winter. For country folk who bathed once a week, that number could add up to a fair crowd lingering outside the door.

Strangely, no one seemed to fault Doc for her arrogance. My father claimed that Doc Hayes knew what his receptionist was doing all along and chose to look the other way. My father felt doctors' employees were extensions of themselves. He told me how doctors hired individuals with similar attitudes and often allowed their employees to convey the messages they didn't have time for or lacked the courage to do themselves. I took this to mean old Doc Hayes was really a bastard, choosing to let his bulldog do his dirty work.

Another twenty minutes passed. The man in the stained overalls had not been called back, nor had I. Easing out of my chair and crossing to where Marge sat now deeply engrossed in *Cosmopolitan*, I tapped on the glass window that separated us.

"What is it, Doctor?"

"I'm leaving," I said. "I have another appointment."

Walking out on Bennington made me feel a shade better. I still had a throbbing shoulder, so I popped two Advil and got back to work.

My next patient was Lacy Timms. Her chart lay on my desk, and on top of it someone had attached a newspaper ad and a yellow sticky note. The advertisement was for Dr. Jerry Phillips. It touted his surgical experience far in excess of my own, even though I was ten years his senior. The note read, "Lacy had laser surgery for her glaucoma by Dr. Phillips two weeks ago."

My last contact with Dr. Phillips had been several years before, when we were seated together at a meeting. He confided in me that his practice was floundering and he didn't know what to do. I gave him my pat answer: if he took good care of his patients, his practice would grow. A month later, his first advertisement appeared in the Dallas newspaper. Initially, I was angry that he had ignored my advice. The longer I thought about it, however, the more I wondered if some blame resided on my shoulders for not reaching out when he asked for help.

In the upper right-hand corner of the advertisement, Dr. Phillips stood beside a laser machine identical to the one I used. The caption read: "Noted eye surgeon brings pioneering technology to the Dallas/ Fort Worth Metroplex." True, it was new technology, but if Phillips was the first surgeon to use the equipment in Dallas, it was not by much. The ad implied that Phillips was the sole provider and had possibly participated in the development of this new laser, which wasn't true.

So why did Dr. Jerry Phillips and a growing group of physicians break with the profession's long tradition against advertising? As they tell it, they were just keeping patients informed about the new and better technologies. What they failed to mention is that these marketing practices dramatically boost their incomes.

Lacy Timms tapped on the front window, her paperwork complete.

"I see you haven't been here for a while," I said, glancing through her chart. I signaled for her to follow me to the examining room.

"Thank you for seeing me." Lacy sounded edgy. She laid out her three-day history of eye pain and redness. "I'm really touchy about my eyes since the surgery."

After a careful examination of her eyes, I pushed away from the microscope. "I think this antibiotic should do it." I handed her a prescription for antibiotic eye drops. "Your pressure seems to be controlled now without drops."

"Thanks to Dr. Phillips."

"I see that you had surgery recently," I said.

A smile spread across Lacy's face. "He operated on one of the Dallas Cowboys. Glaucoma, just like mine."

"That's certainly a strong endorsement."

My insincere comment went right over Lucy's head. "He went to Harvard," she said.

"Who did?"

"Dr. Phillips. It's in the brochure."

"I thought he trained at Kansas," I said.

"A diploma on his wall says Harvard. There's another from Johns Hopkins." Lacy pulled out one of Phillips' brochures from her purse. She pointed to the headline: "Over 900 procedures performed . . ." She said, "He's one of the most experienced doctors in Texas performing this type of surgery. He has a money-back guarantee if my glaucoma doesn't get better."

"Lacy, then why did you come back to me for this problem?"

She looked up at me, her face a picture of contemplation. "I'm embarrassed to say this. But I don't trust him."

Lacy left, and I was alone in my office. I reached for the telephone and dialed the Ophthalmology Department at Southwestern Medical School here in Dallas. Mary Denton, the chairman's secretary, answered.

"Tell me about Jerry Phillips," I said. "I understand he went to Harvard." I knew she kept a current biography on every ophthalmologist who volunteered to help with the teaching program.

"He did," she paused, "for a day. Evidently, Dr. Phillips took a three-hour course on a rare retinal disease, something you might see once every five years. You were invited and probably tossed the invitation with the rest of your junk mail. He attended similar programs at Johns Hopkins and Stanford."

"What about the diplomas?"

"If you mean the certificates. Everyone who attends gets a certificate. Take a look at the fine print."

20

MONEY BACK GUARANTEE

John Stedman barked instructions into his cell phone. He paced around my small examining room and eyed me impatiently. I was running late, and Stedman was irritated. The well-coiffed man in a three-pieced suit slapped the lid to his phone closed and glanced down at the gold Rolex wrapped on his wrist. "Held up on the tenth hole, Doc?"

"I had to stop by the emergency room," I said. A quick scan of his chart told me he was an attorney. "I see you're here for a second opinion. Problems from your LASIK surgery?"

"Disaster would be more like it! Dr. Phillips gave me a guarantee, and he botched the job. I'm going to get my money back and more, if I don't start seeing better."

"Your vision checked out twenty/twenty in each eye."

"I don't give a crap what the chart shows. It's the glare that's blinding me. I'm up at night a lot, running between the hospitals and the jail. The lights are driving me crazy."

"You do most of your work at night?"

"That's when the majority of my clients need my help. During the day, I spend my time in court or taking depositions."

I motioned for him to sit down. Slightly over five minutes passed before I slid away from the examining chair and flipped back on the light. "Not too much there," I said. "Your vision tests out pretty good, but there is a mild haze in both corneas that would explain the glare. Usually it clears over time. I'd consider your results a success."

"They're not your eyes, are they, Doc? Can you make it go away?"

"We can try some topical steroids. There's no assurance the haze will totally clear."

"Phillips screwed up, didn't he? No holding back, Doc. That's what I'm paying you for."

I wanted to say his problem was related to Dr. Phillips questionable marketing practices, but I knew it wasn't. Mr. Stedman and I came from separate disciplines, but we both made our living off medical mishaps. Mr. Stedman had no concept of our differing values.

"The practice of medicine is a profession just like yours, Mr. Stedman. Unlike law, however, it is also a science, based on principles governed by the laws of nature. We have much yet to learn."

"You're like all the other doctors, always covering up for your cronies' mistakes."

"When my father and grandfather were practicing medicine, if a surgical procedure didn't go the way it should, it was called a poor outcome." I stopped, making sure to choose my words carefully. "When the same result occurs today, the first thought that comes to mind is, who screwed up?"

"If doctors would just fess up when they made mistakes, there wouldn't be this problem."

In today's sue-happy climate, Stedman's solution was blatantly disingenuous.

"Almost all those mistakes, as you call them, were errors in judgment or omission. They should be addressed by system changes that assure they don't continue. Virtually none were intentional. But in those rare instances where they were, the infraction should be addressed through the criminal system and not in civil court." I paused to gather my thoughts while I still had Stedman's silence. "Once no criminal intent is proven, we could go to a binding arbitration system where awards are based on actuarial tables for any damages."

Stedman's arms were folded across his chest.

I said, "We could save all the money paid out in contingency fees and pay your cohorts for billable hours."

Stedman looked down at his watch. "Are you going to give me that medicine, doctor? I was due in court ten minutes ago."

"I read in the paper that applications to law school were up 20 percent."

"Everyone wants to be a lawyer these days," he said.

"Ours are down about 10 percent. I guess you can understand why."

It wasn't until late that evening that I realized why Stedman rubbed me the wrong way. It was his insinuation about my being held up on the tenth tee. The remark was meant as a nasty reminder of my tardiness and implied, at least to me, that I was less dedicated than I ought to be. I found his comment distasteful, but not entirely without merit. Many doctors today appear to be less dedicated than previous generations. In my grandfather's era, and even to a certain extent my father's, physicians were literally yoked to their practices. The use of cell phones, e-mail, paperless medical records, and competently staffed emergency departments does not imply that doctors today are any less dedicated, only more in step with advances in technology.

I pulled onto Central Expressway and aimed for the Radisson Hotel. I had a conference to attend, and I was running late. Thunderclouds loomed out to the west and were headed my way. I could only hope the storms would hold off. Otherwise the usual Friday traffic, already inching along, would come to a halt. I noticed a large new billboard up ahead. The words MONEY-BACK GUARANTEE came into focus. The small print at the bottom said "vasectomy reversal" and listed an 800 number.

Scattered showers, the radio said. Trusting the experts, I elected to ignore the rain and stay on the freeway. The small drops quickly grew into a torrent, and I slammed on my brakes, stopping just inches from the car in front of me.

"Damn!"

Meteorology, like medicine, was a science governed by the laws of nature. Despite Doppler radar and the latest computer models, those who devoted their lives to the discipline still couldn't predict outcomes with a hundred-percent accuracy. Meteorologists never offered guarantees, carefully couching their forecasts as predictions.

Likewise, nothing in medicine was a lock, and yet many patients were blinded by a new wave of health care marketing gimmicks. Much of the new marketing minimized the truth—that no surgery is minor, no pill without side effects, and no treatment plan a guarantee. If a particular procedure didn't give the desired results, patients couldn't turn back the clock.

I arrived at the Radisson with enough time to grab a bite from the refreshment table. I loathed the insurance side of my practice, but our group's office manager had laid down the law—we doctors had to do a better job of Medicare coding if we expected to be properly reimbursed. So here I was, away from the office, taking a course in Insurance 101.

It had been a year since I'd last seen my distinguished teacher, Dr. Simpkins, at his retirement reception. Time had not been kind to him. With his hollow cheeks and stooped posture, I barely recognized him.

"Professor," I said. "Are you enjoying your retirement?"

He looked up and splashed coffee from a Styrofoam cup on the floor. "Busier than ever." There was little conviction in his voice. "That's not entirely true. The only thing I'm asked to do anymore is give speeches at retirement ceremonies and eulogies at memorial services. There's not many of us left, you know."

I hoped for a smile, a sign of his dry wit coming through, but there was none. Professor Simpkins had been one of the best teachers I'd ever encountered. His peers considered him one of the patriarchs of radiology, crediting him for raising the specialty to the position of respect it held today. Even as a lowly intern, I remembered his tolerance as I groped my way through the rotation on his service. However, most of his patients probably couldn't recall his name, because—secluded away reading X-rays—he always took second billing to the personal physician. The beauty was that he didn't seem to care. He had a sense of the role his specialty needed to play. He knew how important his part was in helping patients through some of the most trying times in their lives, and that gave him satisfaction. His legacy was that he'd taught the rest of the profession to appreciate that vital role.

He stood before me, his trembling hands gripping the flimsy cup.

"What are you doing here?" I asked.

"Like you, I'm just trying to stay up to date, in case I might want to come out of retirement." It was then he gave me his familiar thin smile. "I've been diagnosed with early Parkinson's disease, but except for the mild trembling, it doesn't seem to have slowed me down."

"I'll bet you still can teach the basics better than anyone."

"You're very kind. But there are rules about retirement. At least, they let me stay on until I turned seventy."

Professor Simpkins drifted into the conference room. I was disheartened that someone with so much to give was wasted on the eulogy circuit.

The conference ran twenty minutes late, and the traffic back to the office was especially heavy. By the time I arrived, my waiting room was abuzz with patients. According to Babs, there were a handful of malcontents. One was Seymour Blevins. Mr. Blevins complained loudly to anyone who would listen.

Once in the exam room, Mr. Blevins said, "My time's as valuable as yours, Doc."

I apologized. "Now, let's see what's going on here."

"You wouldn't refill my eye drops; that's what's going on."

I leafed through his chart. "It was the only way I could get you to come in." Early in my practice, I learned that some patients had to be forced to keep appointments. Reminder cards were sometimes useful, but the thing that kept many of them returning was cutting off their prescription refills. I felt that allowing patients to continue a treatment regimen without monitoring for effectiveness and side effects could sometimes do more harm.

"The last time we saw you was eighteen months ago," I said. "Glaucoma is a serious problem. I hope you've seen a doctor in the meantime."

"No, Doc. I wouldn't trust nobody with these eyes but you. I just had so many things going on. My wife broke her hip, and then the daughter fell out with her husband and moved back in with us."

"The eye drops. Have you been taking them the way I told you?"

"Never miss them." He shifted uneasily in the chair.

"Three times a day. Both eyes?" I asked. If he'd been taking them correctly, he'd have run out of eye drops a long time ago, and we both knew it.

"Yeah, three times."

"Look, Mr. Blevins. There's nothing worse than spending the last part of your life blind. That's what can happen if you don't follow my directions and keep up your appointments. Only you can make that decision. But I don't have to be part of it if you're not willing to try."

"You're being kind of hard on me, Doc." He made no move to leave.

"Here," I said. "A gift from the drug company." I handed him a sample of his eye drops along with a prescription for enough refills to last him three months.

"Thanks, Doc." A smile broke across his face. "I don't want to go blind."

"After you leave here, only you can take care of you."

"Say, Doc, about my time being as valuable as yours, I know you must have had somebody with a real emergency."

"More like a conference that ran late. And bad traffic."

"We all do what we got to do, Doc!" He grinned and headed into the hall. "I'll be sure to make an appointment on the way out."

21

Professional Courtesy

———— ▪ ————

I n the middle of the pastoral prayer, my pager chirped. Echoing off the plastered walls, the sound carried across the massive sanctuary of the Highland Park Presbyterian Church. Janet tried to ignore it, but the others around our church pew craned their necks in my direction. Even the minister looked up and shot a disgruntled stare at me. I quickly slid past two ladies decked out in their Sunday best and pushed through the exit doors.

I made the connection to the long distance number in Waxahachie using the telephone located in the holding area just off the sanctuary.

"Robbie," the voice said. I quickly recognized my caller as Oma Jones, the nurse anesthetist whose cutting remarks during my first visits to the operating room almost thirty years ago had caused me to consider another career. "My eyes feel a little scratchy, and I need to see you. Today."

It had been ten years since I'd heard that voice. I was aware she had undergone cataract surgery earlier this year, but knew nothing more.

"How long have you had the problem?" I asked.

"A week or so." She sounded impatient.

"I heard you recently had your cataracts removed. Did you let the doctor who performed your surgery know about your problem?"

"Oh no! He's a specialist. At Baylor up near you. I didn't want to bother him with something like this."

Even though my father was Harvard trained, I remembered the pain he suffered when some of Waxahachie's finest citizens made the trek to Dallas for their surgeries. His experience taught me a lesson: to some in your hometown, you can never be a hero.

"I'll be glad to work you in tomorrow."

"This is an emergency! I want to be seen today. It's going to take me an hour to get up there."

"I'm afraid tomorrow at eight-thirty is the best I can do."

Oma breathed heavily into the phone. "This isn't the way your daddy would've done business."

My patience was growing thin. I said, "Monday morning, you'll be my first patient."

"Tomorrow's no good for me."

"May I ask why?"

"Robbie," she said, denying me the respect of calling me Doctor, "if you must know, I'm having my teeth cleaned. It took me three weeks to get this appointment. You don't seriously expect me to break it, now do you?"

Oma Jones's eye problem turned out to be a minor infection that, left alone, probably would have cleared on its own. I prescribed a short course of antibiotic drops, probably as much to make me feel better as Oma. When I started to write out the prescription, she balked. Whatever I had in samples would be just fine by her. Oma knew all the angles. I never sent her a bill, and she never sent me a thank you.

Oma Jones never had any intention of paying, but not everyone was like her.

Mrs. Duffy Baltz was a doctor's wife, and my administrative staff had extended her our standard professional courtesy: doctor's wives didn't owe a cent.

"But I want to pay!" she said.

Duffy's husband, Dr. Sidney Baltz, had been a founder of the hospital complex where I now worked. A general surgeon of great distinction, he was one of the first physicians to ask me to care for his family. "If you're Mayo's son, that's good enough for me," he'd said. His remark spoke to the reputation of trust I had inherited based on nothing more than those who had gone before me.

Tragically, Dr. Baltz had sustained irreparable brain damage slightly over five years earlier when he'd been attacked by a junkie scrounging for drugs. Duffy, also his former nurse, never left his side in the ICU until he died from his injury days later.

I watched from down the hall as she rifled through her purse, pulled out some folded bills, and placed the money on the check-out counter. "Take it. Otherwise I won't feel comfortable about coming back." She threw back her shoulders and left the office.

Duffy, like my mother, had spent a lifetime under the protective wing of her husband. Now, faced with his loss, she had a choice: wither away by brooding over her husband's senseless death, or bravely start over. Refusing our offer of professional courtesy was her way of telling us she had chosen to start over.

Not all patients were as demanding as Oma Jones or as willful as Duffy Baltz. Some were simply determined to make the best of whatever challenges came their way.

Betty Marks was one such patient. I first met Betty when I was an intern at Parkland and she was the head nurse on the trauma floor. Even then, she treated me with respect just because I was a doctor. When I began my residency several years later, she sought me out for an eye problem she was having. Even though it turned out to be inconsequential, her gesture of confidence stayed with me. Now she was ravaged by end-stage emphysema and tethered to her lifesaving bottle of oxygen. However, she was no victim.

"Don't you know you're not supposed to ask a girl her age, doctor?" she said.

"It won't go out of this room," I said, needing the information as part of my examination.

"I'm seventy-eight and earned every year of it. You know that from my records you got there." Neatly tucked into a floral scarf knotted around her neck, Betty had an oxygen tube from her nose to an oxygen canister at her side. She glanced at the canister, "*Dammit*, here, and I have been good friends for some time."

"How did your buddy get its name?" I asked.

"Every time I go somewhere, I have to carry him along. I'd say Dammit, let's go, and the name just stuck."

As she told the story, there was still a youthful freshness about her, almost a glow.

One of my medical school professors once opened his presentation with the disturbing observation that we all begin to die the day we are born. He went on to explain that physically, we are at our best somewhere between age eighteen and twenty-eight, pointing out that swimmers and gymnasts are considered old by the time they reach their early twenties and most boxers are past their prime by their early thirties. He then countered these facts by reminding us that when John Kennedy became America's youngest president at forty-three, many people were concerned that he was not mature enough for the job. These examples demonstrated the significant difference between our peak physical and mental ages.

Two years shy of being an octogenarian, Betty embraced the challenges ahead, whereas, many of her counterparts appeared to exist from one illness to the next. To them, aging had become their disease. In Betty's career, she'd probably counseled hundreds of patients about not giving up. It was obvious she had taken her own advice.

The examination completed, Betty reached for her cane and struggled to get out of the chair. She tucked Dammit under one arm and clung to her purse with the other. Even as she fought to right herself, her smile never faded.

"I'll see you next year," she said.

"You know, Betty, you don't seem a day older than when I first started my internship. I'll bet you never will."

As my practice grew, demands on my time grew with it. Those demands meant less time with patients like Oma Jones, Duffy Baltz, and Betty Marks and more time outside the office. I became involved in professional organizations, listened to endless speakers at endless conferences, and even got a chance to lecture myself.

Not long after tending to Betty, I got a call from a good friend and ophthalmology professor. "You'd be doing me a big favor," he said. "It's one lecture, Introduction to Ophthalmology. You'd be addressing the junior class, and we'd be honored to have you. You might even sway a few minds our way."

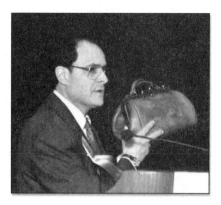

Rob Tenery, MD
Compliments of the Texas Medical Association

Medical school was a long time ago, but with six weeks to prepare for the lecture, I agreed. Medicine had changed since I went through training. Medical students were now forced to choose a career path earlier, especially in the competitive specialties. Some of the most unhappy doctors I've known were those who'd chosen the wrong specialty, one that didn't match their personalities.

When lecture day arrived, I was ready and showed up early. I watched the students trickle in and guessed that out of the class of one hundred and fifty, ten or so might lean toward ophthalmology. Ten minutes after the hour, only twenty or so young faces dotted the large amphitheater.

"Where's the rest of your class?" I asked.

A student straightened up in her chair, looked around. "This should be about it." She reached over and adjusted the volume on a small tape recorder beside her. I'd noticed that several of the students had also brought along tape recorders.

Disappointed at the low turnout, I stumbled into the first part of my lecture. Was the low turnout because I was from the private sector and not a professor with an impressive vitae? Was it the lack of interest in my specialty? I forced myself to stay focused. I presented the information in straightforward fashion, brought up the lights, and began what I assumed would be a plodding question-and-answer session. I was wrong. The students threw questions at me until long past my time allotment.

A week later, I got a call from the ophthalmology professor thanking me for filling in.

"I'm not sure you made the right decision," I said, "asking me to stand in. Only twenty or so students showed up."

"That's almost ten more than I got last year." The professor sounded amused at my concern. "The students use note services. I rarely get over a couple of dozen students in any given lecture. Instead of attending class, they use note services to take down the information, label and organize it so it's easy to reference, and distribute the notes. The students form study groups and divvy up the other work: reading, research, whatever. Most of the class participates in group assignments."

"It sounds like students miss a lot of class," I said.

"They claim it's more efficient this way. The information is organized and easy to memorize. Still, it's not perfect. Except for what they do in the labs, students aren't actively participating. There's very little direct feedback."

What a difference from my own days, where I sat frozen in my seat for hours scribbling fact after fact as the professors rattled on. I'd been a note-taking machine and hadn't much liked it. Maybe the note services were an improvement. Yet, I remembered how one of my anatomy professors, the colorful Raymond Mount, taught us the anatomy of the small intestine by climbing atop his marble-topped lectern and wrapping himself in toilet paper. How would that memorable moment have been captured by a note service?

■ ■

About a week after my lecture at the medical school, a patient asked me to speak with her son. My patient, Mrs. Raney, wanted me to dazzle her son with the ins and outs of the medical profession.

The son, Josh, was unkempt with shaggy hair and a gold stud through his eyebrow.

"Nice digs you have here," he said, referring to my office.

"My wife did the decorating," I said. "Your mother tells me you're thinking about becoming a doctor."

"Among other things." He pulled out a legal pad from a dingy backpack. "One of my professors told me the future is like a fruit basket with a lot of choices. We have to be careful to pick the right one."

"I agree with your professor. How about I start with why I became a doctor, and then you—"

"Sorry to interrupt. I know you're busy, doctor. Why don't we make it more efficient for both of us and let me ask a few questions I've written down here."

"This sort of feels like a deposition," I said in half-jest.

"Exactly. Here we go. One government mandate after another tells doctors, you, how to practice. Am I right?"

"Yes and no—"

"Hold on. The way I see it, doctors are giving up high-risk procedures because of the rising cost of malpractice premiums."

"Or moving to states where the premiums aren't as high."

"Exactly. And no one cares. Political leaders won't help, patient groups like AARP aren't on your side, and I don't think I even have to mention the media."

"You've noticed." I was impressed at his grasp of the issues facing medicine. "Medicine isn't what it used to be, but—"

He cut me off. Again. "Before coming to see you, I borrowed a white coat from my sister's boyfriend, who works for a lab over at Presbyterian Hospital." He pointed to the white bundle wadded under his backpack. "I slipped into the doctors' dining room here at Medical City. My professor said this was the best way to get the pulse. You know, what's really going on."

I was a little taken aback by his directness. "And?" I said.

"I can tell you, the mood wasn't good. Many of your colleagues are griping about working harder, taking home less money. That sort of thing."

"I suspect that's true of most professions. Sure, a lot of doctors are dissatisfied with their practices, but—"

Josh stuffed his legal pad into his backpack. He straightened, looked at me, and raised the eyebrow with the gold stud in it. The motion looked practiced to me. "Kids my age, college students, not too many are choosing medicine. What's happening to your profession, doctor?"

I wanted to say to Josh, "With all due respect, you're right. We've got problems you can't begin to imagine. But that doesn't make your flippant attitude, abrasive habit of interrupting, and ridiculous choice of personal adornment any easier to swallow." I didn't say any of that. What I said was, "Josh, your concerns are correct. However, you've failed to evaluate the three most important aspects of being a doctor: First, job security. There would always be a need for doctors. Second, the respect and recognition we receive from our patients. Third, the personal satisfaction that comes from helping others through some of the most difficult times in their lives."

"That's all well and good, doctor. But, I just don't know." Josh picked up his backpack and climbed out of the chair. "Most doctors are close to thirty before they start earning a living. I'm not sure it's for me."

Following Josh to the door, I knew he had already made his decision.

22

SURROGATES ARE NOT QUITE THE SAME

In late spring, a high school friend, Dave, was admitted to the hospital here at Medical City. First thing the next morning, I looked in on him. He told me he hadn't seen his doctor since his admission.

"What do you mean?" I asked.

"Just that. I haven't seen him. There have been a lot of doctors in and out of here, but not mine." Dave lay in bed on the fifth floor. "When I asked the nurse what was wrong with me, she said I'd have to talk to Dr. Snavely."

I felt a pang of guilt. Dave had been seeing his long-time general practitioner, Doc Bagley, in Waxahachie. He had a low-grade fever and a lingering malaise. After a battery of tests, Doc Bagley still hadn't been able to come up with a diagnosis. So I'd convinced Dave to come here and see Dr. Snavely. Ron Snavely and I had several mutual patients, yet we hadn't met. When I called to arrange Dave's appointment, I never got past Snavely's nurse. She agreed to squeeze Dave in at the end of the week.

A young woman popped her head in the room. "Excuse me. I'm, Laura, Dr. Snavely's PA. I wanted to ask if there's anything I can do for you while we're waiting for your test results."

I felt like an outsider as the two conversed, Dave from his bed and Laura partially hidden behind the door. Laura wasn't a nurse or

a technician, but a physician's assistant. Supposedly, her job was to
weed through the routine problems so Snavely could spend his time
on more serious matters.

"When will Dr. Snavely be here?" Dave asked.

Her face tightened. "He's very busy. I'm sure when we find out
something, he'll let you and your general practitioner . . ." She pulled a
card from her pocket. "That's Doctor Bagley in Waxahachie, isn't it?"
Laura gave us an embarrassed grin and shuffled into the hall, off to
see her next patient.

"She was the one I saw in the office before I was admitted," Dave said.

"What did Snavely have to say?"

"I never saw him." He shook his head again. "What's he like, anyway?"

"He's ah . . ." I paused, realizing I'd never met the man. In fact, the
more I thought about it, I'd never talked to him. I'd spoken to his
nurse several times. "He has a great reputation," I said.

"Did I ever tell you Doc Bagley delivered me? Then on my birthday,
when I broke my arm, it was Doc who put it in a cast." Dave had a
frown on his face. "When I decided to get married, who do you think
I talked to about planned parenthood? And you don't have to guess
who delivered both our children. The old Doc even came all the way
to Dallas to visit my father after he had bypass surgery."

"And pallbearer, I remember, at your dad's funeral."

Dave nodded. "He's always been there for me and my family."

In the silence of Dave's hospital room, I think both Dave and I
wanted Dr. Snavely to be another Doc Bagley. Although the faces
would change, the need for that relationship did not.

Laura, the PA, burst into the room. "Good news! Dr. Snavely feels
you have infectious mononucleosis. With bed rest for the next couple
of weeks and these medicines, you should be fine." She laid several
prescriptions on the bedside stand. "I'll fill out your discharge papers
and get Dr. Snavely to sign them."

"That's it?" Dave pushed himself upright. "I've never even seen this
guy Snavely."

"I thought you'd be pleased," she said.

"Well I'm not. I came here to see a specialist. I asked my friend here
for his advice, and he said this was the place. But did I actually see a
specialist? No, I didn't."

"Dr. Snavely is very busy," Laura said.

"I know plenty about being busy," Dave said. "For several years, I've been busy developing applications for telemedicine, where medical information is transferred by the telephone. So, I know something about doctors trying to help people out in stretches of West Texas where there are no doctors." Dave glared at Laura. "But this ain't West Texas."

Laura, the PA, glanced at her watch, said she had somewhere to be, and that was the end of the conversation. I walked Dave to his car, and we said our good-byes. In some ways, I think I felt worse than Dave. I'd encouraged him to come here. "This is the place," I'd said. "We have the facilities. We have the talent." And what did he get for his effort? A prescription and a recommendation for bed rest from a well-intentioned surrogate.

When I got back to the office, I noticed a yellow sticky on my exam-room door. It was from Dr. Snavely. I returned the call. The nurse on the patient's floor told me that Dr. Snavely had left an order for me to consult with a patient, Karen Brown, in room 607.

Hospital consults had always been a pet peeve of mine. Being asked to see someone not already part of my planned schedule was an imposition. If I needed to do the evaluation in the hospital room, it was even more trying. I was still upset with Dr. Snavely. I also resented the way his request was delivered. It came across as a demand.

"What's the problem, exactly?" I asked the nurse over the telephone.

"I don't know. He just wanted you to see the patient."

"I don't do consults without talking to the doctor first."

"I can give you Dr. Snavely's number," the nurse said.

"Tell Dr. Snavely that if he wants me to see his patient, he needs to call me."

"But, he wants you to—"

"Please, have him call me."

I got the call five minutes later. Only it wasn't Dr. Snavely on the phone. It was Laura, the PA. She said, "Karen Brown is a thirty-year-old female who was admitted to the hospital for a workup of fever of unknown etiology." Her straight-to-the-point delivery reminded me of the computeresque voice on the weather station. "Dr. Snavely wants you to perform a retinal evaluation."

Since the internal landscape of the eye often reveals signs of systemic medical conditions, Snavely's request was not uncommon for patients with a questionable medical diagnosis. Most of the physicians give me a heads-up regarding the potential list of maladies. Not Dr. Snavely. His request would send me on a scavenger hunt with no clues.

"What does he suspect?" I asked.

"We just admitted her, so I don't have that information."

"Has Dr. Snavely seen the patient?"

"I did her physical in the office and—"

"Once Dr. Snavely has examined his patient, have him call me."

Later that afternoon, Dr. Snavely returned my call. He was vague about his findings and had no more information than Laura the PA.

I grabbed my examination paraphernalia and made my way over to the hospital. Karen Brown's room lay in muted darkness.

"Dr. Snavely?" she asked. "What's happening to me?"

"I'm the eye doctor. Dr. Snavely has asked me to take a look at you."

"You're not Dr. Snavely?" Karen shivered under the mound of white blankets. "I'm so cold."

"Dr. Snavely will be along later." I hoped that Snavely wouldn't prove me a liar. "Now, tell me how this all started."

Back at the nurse's station, I scribbled my findings on Karen Brown's chart. She had one isolated hemorrhage near her left optic nerve and yellowing of her conjunctiva, suggesting early jaundice. Other than that, I wasn't able to add much to the search for the cause of her condition.

Passing Karen's darkened room on my way to the elevator, I realized how vulnerable patients become on the far end of the stethoscope. Unless told otherwise, they are left to imagine the worst. It's often the physician's bedside manner that separates the good doctors from the great ones. How doctors relate to their patients isn't a part of the medical school curriculum. Even if it were, I've discovered that compassion can only come from within. As many physicians raise their technical skills to new levels, the solace they show their patients is often subjugated to science.

I'd barely reached my office when the back phone lit up.

Dr. Snavely said, "That patient in 607 turns out to have infectious hepatitis. Her liver profile just came through. I'll have Laura tell her. If she takes care of herself, she should get through it."

"Why don't you tell her yourself," I said.

"I've got other patients to tend to."

"We all have other patients. This one needs you. Now."

"Who do you think you are?"

A long pause followed. Controlling my anger, I said, "Go on over and talk to her. Five minutes."

"I guess I could."

"The patient in 607," I said. "Her name is Karen Brown."

How Dr. Snavely handled the situation with Karen Brown, I'd never know. Would he avoid her? Was she just another room number, unworthy of his personal attention? Or did he feel uncomfortable in one-to-one situations? Some of the best minds in our profession are poor communicators. As medical students, we used to refer to them as professorial types, since many sought refuge in academic laboratories where they wouldn't see patients. Others become super-specialists, raising their level of expertise in some narrow field so there was no one left to question them, including their patients.

I recalled seeing one of Dr. Snavely's patients, Ray, in my office several weeks earlier. In his late fifties, with a disconcerting hand tremor, Ray had been referred to me for a baseline examination before starting on a new, potentially toxic medication. When I asked what he was being treated for, his answer was surprisingly vague.

"Dr. Snavely didn't really tell me, Doc. He's a good doctor. One of the best, I'm told. With all those patients, I guess he's just too busy to explain it all."

Now, weeks later, I wondered how Ray was doing with the new medication. What happened if Dr. Snavely was wrong? Would Ray still think his good doctor was all that good? Medicine is an inexact science. Without a relationship based on caring, doctors who fail to communicate must rely on how their patients respond to treatment. If a particular patient does well, the physician's lack of bedside manner is excused. If the patient does poorly, questions are often raised.

In my grandfather's day, patients were so thankful for any medical help that they rarely asked questions. Many patients thought doctors were omniscient. They were afraid to ask questions and suspected they couldn't understand the answers if they did. Today the media exploits the slightest infraction, and our legal system blurs the line between poor outcomes and negligence. By failing to communicate with patients, the Dr. Snavelys of our profession put themselves at risk. Worse, patients are left to trust in their doctors' skills and not in their hearts.

23

THE HEALTH CARE PAYMENT DILEMMA

I t was late September on a Sunday afternoon when I received a call from the emergency room in Mesquite where my partners and I ran a satellite office. The young resident working there gave me the summary information. A girl had dived into a lake headfirst and hit the bottom.

"The blow shoved her eye back in her head," he said. "I don't think she knew how low the lake was."

Summers in Central Texas are dry. Most of the lakes are man-made, created as reservoirs for the surrounding water districts. As the summer droughts linger, the surrounding communities continue to suck out their quota of water to feed the lawns, pools, and bathtubs. What are left are puddles where the lake used to be. Most Texans abandon the lakes by late August. A few diehards still use them, often tearing up their boats on the tree stumps and sand bars. Some, tragically, end up with head and neck injuries when they misjudge the lakes' shallow bottoms.

"She'll need more than an ophthalmologist," I said. "Why don't you evacuate her to Medical City, where I can call in a neurosurgeon?"

"I'd hoped that's what you'd say. Someone from administration will notify Medical City that you're willing to accept the patient, and then I'll arrange the transfer."

"Go ahead and send for the ambulance. I'll make the calls."

Within minutes, I had spoken with one of Medical City's assistant administrators, who agreed to accept the patient. I left out one important piece of information, however: the patient's insurance coverage. When I worked at the hospital in Waxahachie, whether or not patients had coverage was never a question. Medicine was now big business, and if the health care institutions wanted to keep their doors open, they had no choice but to pay attention to the bottom line.

I dialed back the resident, but he was busy. I asked for the nurse on duty. "She's tied up helping Dr. Blake. If you're calling about the patient we've transferred to your hospital, the ambulance picked her up ten minutes ago."

I could only hope the patient's insurance coverage would not prove a problem.

An hour later, I received a call. "Your patient has arrived, doctor."

When I reached the emergency room, I came face to face with the assistant administrator, a clipboard in her hand. "Did you know your patient has no insurance?" she said.

"No, I didn't," I said. "I tried to call the hospital, but I didn't connect with anyone."

"You should have gotten that information before we accepted this patient."

"Can we do this another time?" I called to the nurse standing behind the administrator. "Where did they put my patient?"

I disappeared into the examining room. After a quick evaluation, I realized the patient had ruptured her right eye and the X-ray on the view box revealed a part of her skull was dislodged into her cranial cavity. "Who's on neurosurgery call?"

The nurse removed a sheet of paper from her pocket. "Dr. Mahon."

Dr. Mahon and I had both trained at Parkland Hospital. I was an intern two months out of medical school, and Mahon was the chief resident in neurosurgery. Although the encounter was almost twenty years ago, it was one I would never forget. Paramedics had brought in a man in a coma. They'd found him in an alley where they'd assumed he had been living. The emergency room was busy that night, and they'd placed him in one of the trauma rooms before charging off to the next emergency. It was the very room where President Kennedy had spent his final moments after he had been shot. Due to a screw-up with the crew change, the man had been forgotten. When I arrived at seven o'clock a.m., I pushed open the door to the trauma room and discovered the patient choking on his own vomit. I was able to clear his airway and insert an endotracheal tube.

Dr. Mahon blasted into the ER. "Where's my coma patient?"

I pointed to the trauma room. "Room one. I just saved his life."

Dr. Mahon rushed past me into the room. He returned moments later. "You did call for radiology? We need an arteriogram."

"I just found him."

"Did you make the call or not?"

"It didn't occur to me."

"I'll do it myself."

Dr. Mahon and I had ended up practicing in the same institution, and our first encounter never came up. Although I assumed his recollection of the event had faded long ago, mine had not. I felt embarrassed, and the memory had stayed with me all these years.

I asked the nurse, "Would you please page Dr. Mahon and ask him to help me with this patient?"

With the patient's vital signs worsening, we had to move quickly. The young woman was moved to the operating room suite, where I sutured her ruptured eye. Dr. Mahon arrived and performed a four-hour surgery to put her skull back in position. We hardly spoke. After completing my part of the surgery, I did manage to get in a thank you. He gave me a brief nod.

Late the next afternoon Dr. Mahon showed up at my office. "Doctor," he said.

I rose from my desk braced for his verbal onslaught. "Before you begin, I didn't know she was uninsured." Dr. Mahon's permanent frown reminded me of my grandfather.

"That's not why I'm here."

"Insured or not, the woman needed our help."

He leaned against the door jamb. "Any time you have a patient that needs my help, don't worry whether they can pay or not."

The patient made it through surgery and was transferred to Parkland

Hospital for rehabilitation. Medical City had shouldered the burden of the cost of her surgeries. Now it was time for the citizens of Dallas County to do their part.

——— ▪ ———

Three weeks later, long-time patient Mary Potter made an appointment with me for the sole purpose of asking me to help her find another doctor. Her health insurance company had recently changed, and one of the new company's requirements was to pick an eye doctor from the company's list of participating physicians. Miss Potter handed me the physician listing brochure.

"I hate to do this," Mary said. "But can you tell me who to choose?"

I took the list and underlined several ophthalmologists. "Any of these doctors will take good care of you."

"No one knows me like you do, doctor."

A pang of remorse tugged at me. When Mary was six, her mother brought her to me. At the time, the other kids in Mary's kindergarten class teased her because she had one badly crossed eye. The same eye had a cataract, making it look cloudy and opaque. Mary's mother, a devout Christian Scientist, had experienced a difficult delivery, and the resulting trauma had left Mary disfigured. Her parents' religious beliefs prevented them from seeking medical care for her eyes until the ridicule got so bad Mary couldn't take it. Although her vision in the injured eye would never be clear, after two surgeries to straighten her eye and remove her cataract, Mary looked normal, and the ridicule stopped.

"Let me get a copy of your records," I said. "Have your new doctor contact me anytime."

I was beginning to sound like the insurance company, my reactions both formulaic and devoid of emotion. To think that everything doctors knew about their patients was chronicled in the charts was ridiculous.

Many people decry the authority assumed by today's health insurance companies, but it was not unexpected. My father once said, "With all the scientific breakthroughs, and the cost of those discoveries, one day this country will not be able to offer everything to everyone. There's only so much money we have to spend for health care. When we exceed that number, some system will have to decide who gets what."

He'd thought it would be the federal government, as in Canada and England. With the growth of the federal Medicare and Medicaid programs, his fears about government-mandated medical care were partially realized. However, it was managed care, introduced when large businesses sought relief for the high cost of health insurance for employees, that tipped the balance of power to the payer. New technology made going without insurance unthinkable for anyone who could afford the premiums.

Mary had no choice. Either she found a new set of doctors, went to the hospitals listed in her book, and took the medicines printed in her drug formulary, or she faced the possibility of filing for bankruptcy if she ever came down with a major illness or injury. I stood up to shake Mary's hand. Instead, she grabbed me around the chest and pulled me to her. "Can I call if I really need you?"

I realized that even though I was not on Mary's insurance, I would always be her doctor.

———— ■ ————

Thursday morning started out all wrong. One of the technicians who normally helped me work up patients called in with a bad case of tourista. The other arrived twenty minutes late. An elderly couple from Waxahachie appeared at the front window two days ahead of schedule and refused to make the trip back home without a prescription for new glasses. An hour into the day, I was already two hours behind schedule. When the call came in from Dr. Kiltz, it sent my pulse up another ten beats.

"Dr. Kiltz is on hold for you." Babs said. "It sounds urgent."

I slipped out of the exam room and took the phone. "Yes," I said, "Dr. Kiltz?"

"Dr. Kiltz is in with a patient, doctor," answered a voice. "I'll let him know you're available."

Minutes later an unfamiliar voice said, "Bob, Johnny Kiltz here."

I cringed. "I'm sorry, but I don't recognize your name."

He cut me off. "Moved in with Reeves on the second floor a month ago. I'm doing the kidney transplants around here now that my partner's decided to give up some of the hard stuff. That isn't what I called about."

"Welcome to the hospital. How can I help?"

"Contact lenses. Everyone tells me you're the expert around here. What do you think of them? "

"Well, I fit them, and I wear them myself."

"Bob, I've got a break in my schedule around noon. I wonder if you could squeeze me in, so I could try on a pair."

It didn't take long to size up Kiltz as one of those who thinks the world rotates around him.

"Johnny, let me check with my receptionist to see what she has scheduled for me during my lunch break." I punched the button without giving him a chance to reply. It was a good five minutes before I got back on the line. "Sorry, but you know how hectic it can get around here."

"Yeah, sure," he said.

"I've got a previous lunchtime meeting, but we can work you in. Since you'll be doing the kidney transplants around here, we want you to see well, Johnny."

"That would be great."

"Monday, the fifteenth, at eight-thirty."

There was a pause on the other end of the line. "Bob, that's over three weeks away."

"The contacts will be worth the wait. We don't want to rush you through. You'll be here about two hours. So be sure to book enough time out of the office."

Bertha Palmer suffered from elevated intraocular pressure, early changes in her visual fields, and a family history of blindness from the disease. The diagnosis of glaucoma was clear-cut. I'd caught her problem early, and with the proper treatment, she would do well. No matter how hard I try, some patients seem deaf to my instructions and possibly to the world around them. Bertha was one of them.

In medical school, we learned about "White Coat Syndrome," a phenomenon in which a patient experiences extreme anxiety around a doctor. I felt Mrs. Palmer should have passed that barrier long ago.

Several days after her last visit, I received a call from Mrs. Palmer's son.

"My mother didn't hear a word you told her, doctor," he said. "When you mentioned glaucoma, I guess she just shut down."

I scanned Mrs. Palmer's chart, then laid out the facts of his mother's problem as concisely as possible. He thanked me and hung up. I leafed through Bertha Palmer's record one more time. In hindsight, I realized it wasn't what I had said to Mrs. Palmer, but what I hadn't. I'd given her the facts: her intraocular pressures, early changes in her visual fields, and an outline of how glaucoma ran in families. I piled facts on facts, never once addressing her worst fear: ending up blind like her mother.

What I failed to realize was that Mrs. Palmer didn't need or want all the facts. What she needed was assurance that with proper treatment she wouldn't go blind. My job was to sort through the facts, come up with the proper diagnosis, and present it to her in such a way she could cope with her problem. I had failed.

I'd failed because I was focusing on the diagnosis and not the person. Without realizing it, I'd made Mrs. Palmer into another case of glaucoma, instead of a person with glaucoma. My grandfather once told me not to ever forget that there was a patient and not an illness under the sheets. "They only listen when you're talking to them," he said.

I punched in Mrs. Palmer's telephone number.

24

OLD SCHOOL

━━━━━ ∎ ━━━━━

I scanned the advertisement I'd cut from the newspaper. The headline read: "Would you trust your eyes to anyone but the best?" The article described how Dr. Peter Laird, a young ophthalmologist who set up his practice about two years ago near Medical City, was celebrating the Memorial Day weekend by offering a $500 discount to the first twenty veterans seeking LASIK vision correction. In addition, Peter would make a donation to the Veterans of Foreign Wars' charity on behalf of these individuals as a token of his appreciation for their dedication. A footnote said that he was offering a $200 discount to a spouse and one friend, if accompanied by a veteran.

The ad was disingenuous at best. I stuffed the piece of paper in my pocket, hung my shirt inside my locker, and then slipped into my scrubs.

Peter hurried into the doctors' dressing room. "I see you got four on the schedule for this morning."

Peter frequently helped out Dr. Lane Bradley on Tuesdays with his heavy case load. Bradley, who also relied heavily on advertising, usually scheduled twenty or more surgeries a day and was probably grateful for Dr. Laird's assistance.

"My usual," I said. "Maybe I'm doing something wrong."

"You're old school, that's all." He took on a serious look. "Rob, it's unfortunate, but these days you have to get your name out there if you plan to make a living."

I pulled the article from my locker and waved it in Peter's direction. "Ever been in the military, Peter?"

"Look, I'm doing these guys a favor. I give them a discount and everyone goes home happy. The whole veterans' thing was my publicist's idea. Do a little advertising, get some name recognition, and I pick up a few patients." Peter paused. "My family and I have done without for a long time. Take a look at Bradley. This guy bought a house on Jasper Lane, and he's doubling its size. He drives a Mercedes 500SE. Six months ago, my wife and I drove a ten-year-old Nissan. I tried it without advertising." A hint of remorse, barely detectable. "I really did. It didn't work. With all the optometrists and new ophthalmologists in town, it just takes too long to get established. I do a little advertising, and look what happens."

"So what happens?" I asked.

"We're moving to a larger home nearer the country club. And if you hadn't noticed, that red Porsche in the parking lot, it's mine."

"Does it matter what other doctors think?"

"Depends on the doctors. Your generation or mine? Doctors like Bradley, sure I care. In fact, he's not happy with me; I trumped him on the veterans' discount." Peter pulled up his scrub pants and headed for the door. "I have to run. I promised Bradley I'd do a couple of cases for him until he got here. He's attending a board meeting for one of his charities."

"Bradley's not doing his own cases?"

"Hell, the patient's are half-asleep. As long as they get results, they don't care." He pulled back the door and looked over at me. "I know what you're thinking, and it's old school. These patients don't want us to hold their hand. They want us to improve their vision."

Maybe Dr. Peter Laird was right: I was old school. But he was dead wrong about patients' attitudes. To my father, being a doctor was all about trust. He told me he'd seen that trust in the faces of fellow soldiers. He'd seen the same thing in German prisoners in the hospital during World War II. My father was the enemy before they were captured. After, he was their doctor. They had to trust him. Just as important, he wouldn't do anything to betray that trust.

Though he was never critical of doctors who drove Cadillacs, my father never did. He didn't want to project an image of affluence when many of his patients lived from crop to crop. In his final years, as he watched the transfer of power from his generation of doctors to mine, he'd grown more tolerant. He told me once that I shouldn't feel guilty if I wanted to drive a fancy car or wear a custom-fitted suit, if that's what made me happy. He was adamant about one point: don't ever let your patients question your motivation.

Several days later, Janet and I had dinner with her father. Pushing aside the tray of oysters, he held out his hand and said, "This finger of mine, it's lost all its strength."

I leaned closer, the loud music making it hard to hear. "Well, you just had surgery a month ago. It takes a while." I tried to reassure him that his recovery was going well. The surgery was to repair the sheath around a tendon in his index finger. Commonly called "trigger finger," the finger becomes swollen and is often painful to straighten once bent. "What does your doctor say about your progress?"

"This is the God's truth," he said. "Except for the two minutes I saw him in the office when he first examined me, I haven't laid eyes on him. Even then, he didn't talk to me. He spoke some sort of doctor code to his nurse, telling her what was wrong with me, to get me scheduled for surgery as soon as possible, and some other things I didn't catch."

Papa Joe's doctor, Sterling Freeman, had an outstanding reputation. Although I'd never met the man, I'd heard glowing reports about his surgical skills. So I was surprised at my father-in-law's experience.

"What about before surgery?" I asked.

"The anesthesiologist had me asleep so quick I never saw him. Afterward, Freeman's nurse saw me and did the discharge. For all I know, someone else could have done the operation. When I went back to get my stitches out, I could hear his voice off in some other part of the office, but he never came in to personally check me." He awkwardly placed his cup on the table. "I know he's supposed to be the best, but I'd like a chance to ask him a few questions."

Freeman sounded like another Snavely.

"Just give his office a call and tell them you want to talk to him, personally."

"I tried. Even gave the receptionist the questions in advance. His nurse returned my call with what she claimed were his answers. She said he was tied up in surgery." Papa Joe gazed across the busy restaurant and clenched his fist several times. "As long as I continue to improve, I guess it's okay."

"Are you going back if you don't get better?"

He shook his head. "I don't know."

I thought of Lane Bradley, who skipped surgery if he had other obligations. And Snavely, who used Laura, a physician's assistant, as his extension. And now Freeman, whose face was known only to a select few. These physicians came from different eras and disciplines, yet they had one thing in common: they based their practices on results, and not on relationships.

Josie Chapman had come to me for a second opinion.

"I just don't know what to do," she said. "I was at the park over by my house last weekend with my grandkids when this nice young man tells me he can check my eyes for free. He was working out of a van with Dr. Bradley's name painted on the side in large letters. I wasn't the only one. He was checking other people there too. So, I climb inside and, after he shines all these lights in my eyes, he tells me I need surgery for my cataracts."

"Were you aware that you had cataracts?" I asked.

"No sir. I thought my eyes were healthy. I sing in the choir every Sunday, and I can see everybody, even those on the back pew."

Her vision was only one line below normal. "Did the technician suggest you try a change in your glasses first?"

She shook her head. "No sir, not that I recall. Only that they would send a limousine to pick me up for surgery on Wednesday and take me back home after." She broke into a smile. "I've never been in a limousine."

Under the guise of bringing better care, Dr. Lane Bradley had dispatched one of his technicians to screen for disease among the less advantaged. Bradley may have been concerned about identifying undetected problems, but I suspected he was more interested in gathering candidates for surgery, a practice called "trolling" in medical circles.

After completing my evaluation, I flipped on the light. "Josie, you do have cataracts, but it may be years until you need to have them removed. What did you say to Dr. Bradley's technician about the surgery on Wednesday?"

She squinted as her eyes adjusted to the light. "They asked me for my address and I gave it to them."

"Even though you didn't feel you had a problem?"

Josie folded her hand in her lap. "I thought we were supposed to trust doctas to do right by us."

Bradley's actions reflected negatively on the whole of the profession. Not only was he squandering the trust he inherited from past generations of physicians, but he was violating the law. Medicare and the other health care payers have precise criteria for cataract surgery. Josie Chapman didn't meet any of those criteria. Her early-stage cataracts didn't impede her life. Her vision was only one line less than perfect.

She asked. "So what should I do?"

"On Wednesday, when they come to pick you up, I wouldn't answer the door."

25

The Power of Commitment

Some doctors were old school. Others were old, *old* school.

Dr. Phil Green was a flawless example. Phil was an orthopedic surgeon five years my senior and the embodiment of traditional values like trust, credibility, and commitment. A year or so earlier, he had been accidently infected with hepatitis B from an inadvertent needle stick during surgery. With the disease ravaging his body, he had quit attending our county medical society meetings and undergone a liver transplant.

Martin Both, associate executive for the county medical society, had suggested Phil for a committee I was on, and he wanted my opinion.

Both said, "I think Phil would be perfect for this appointment. But with his recent surgery, I don't know if he's up to it."

I said, "The surgery was only five months ago."

"That's not a long time."

"The worst he could say is no."

"Do you mind making the call?"

I phoned Phil, got him on the line, and stammered out the invitation. "Martin and I were wondering, well, if you'd consider joining our committee. We'd understand if you said no. You've been through a lot."

I'd probably have responded with a quick "no thanks." But Phil didn't. He said, "I'll do it!"

Weeks later, returning from the American Medical Association's meeting in Chicago, we were on a flight to Dallas. We'd gotten the roomier seats just behind the bulkhead. Karen, Phil's wife, and Janet were in the row behind us. I sipped my Coke as we waited for the meal.

Phil reached over and patted my arm. "If I can save just one life, it will be worth the effort."

At the meeting, Phil had championed a controversial resolution to undertake a study to increase the number of organs donated for transplantation. He'd testified before the raucous crowd, citing his own lifesaving experience, and swayed enough votes to pass the resolution.

Now Phil said, "Without the surgery, I wouldn't have been able to walk my daughter down the aisle or shoot that hole-in-one two months ago. My baby granddaughter, I'd've never held her in my hands." Tears filled my eyes. "My liver was a gift," he said. "The young woman who died didn't make this donation so that I could squander my life."

I knew from his speech that 30 percent of people waiting for a liver transplant die before they get one. Almost half of all children who need an organ die because there aren't enough to go around. At the same time, according to Phil, "We bury enough transplantable organs each year to cut the waiting list in half."

If my father had been able to hold out a few years longer, he might have been a candidate for a lung transplant.

I said, "Do you think the AMA's resolution will make a difference?"

"Next week is my liver's second birthday." He squeezed my arm, hard. "The donor's parents entrusted me with the most important thing they had to give—a second chance." Phil reached in his jacket pocket. "Have you filled out a donation card lately?"

"I'm not sure. I think it's on my driver's license."

"They did away with that years ago."

"Then I'm not a donor." I suddenly felt guilty for not being more aware.

"You're not a donor, but you'd be willing to be a recipient if your life was on the line?" He handed me the small stack of cards with Organ

Donor imprinted across the top. "Take these and pass them around. Keep one for yourself."

⸻ ■ ⸻

In the spirit of doing my part for donor transplantation, I accepted an invitation I might otherwise have turned down. The ophthalmology department at the medical school had decided that the practice of having its residents retrieve eyes for corneal transplantation was an inefficient use of time. Morticians were the logical next choice. They were in close contact with the body and they were trained at restorative skills. First, they had to be taught a procedure called enucleation. My job, once I accepted the invitation, was to help train budding morticians at the Dallas Mortuary Academy how to remove the eye, while leaving the remaining orbital contents intact.

When I arrived at the Academy, I had an uneasy feeling in my stomach. I tried to reassure myself that I was just supposed to lecture on the procedure. The eye removal process wasn't difficult as long as one was familiar with anatomy. It was just a matter of clipping a few muscles and severing the optic nerve. The first couple of times I was nervous, but it didn't take long to become routine. How the Academy came up with my name, I'll never know. My guess is, I was the first to say yes.

I have never been much for cadavers. Even during the anatomy course in my first year of medical school, I'd never gotten over that edgy feeling. Although many of my classmates would stay late into the night meticulously dissecting every nerve and vessel, I relied more on learning from the color diagrams in the anatomy atlas. During my ophthalmology residency, I was once again forced to be around cadavers, or more accurately, the recently deceased, before they were embalmed. Removing their eyes took me to some very unsettling places, from the county morgue to the basements of funeral homes, usually in the middle of the night. It was the one thing that made me question my decision to go into ophthalmology. When the request came in from the mortuary school, I agreed in part to spare future residents from this distasteful duty.

A man in the stained butcher's apron opened the door and ushered me in to Classroom 103. "Good to see you, doctor." I wrinkled my nose at the irritating smell of glycerine laced with formaldehyde. Approximately thirty students mingled in small groups at the back of the room. "You're just in time," he said, "I'm Professor Graves."

Letting the irony of his last name slide, I recognized the rectangular table at the front of the small lecture hall from my old anatomy days at medical school. Atop the table, covered with a canvas sheet, was the silhouette of a human body. I extended my hand.

"Break's over," he said and moved toward the front of the class. "The doctor is here to teach you how to snatch out eyes."

"It's called enucleation," I said under my breath. Fumbling with the binder containing my lecture notes, I looked around for the lectern. "Professor, where do I put my notes?"

The professor's eyes darted from side to side and then lit on the lumpy mound in front of him. "Doctor, I guess this will just have to do." He pointed to the corpse on the table.

All eyes in the room locked onto me as I tried to find just the right place on the cadaver to balance the binder.

My presentation took all of twenty minutes.

As I stepped away from the table to accept the audience's applause, Professor Graves moved to my side. His fingers were clasped around several surgical instruments.

"Doctor, the class and I have one final request." He stripped back the canvas cover to expose the cadaver's head. "We would be honored if you would give us a demonstration of your enucleation technique. After, if you have the time, we'll treat you to lunch in our cafeteria."

———————— ▬ ▪ ▬ ————————

Walking down the hallway to the examining room, Beulah Pennington wore shiny new glasses as thick as Coke bottles. Her patterned dress could have been made from a flour sack. The bonnet hiding the furrows in her aging brow was straight out of an old Sears catalogue. One hand was wrapped around the head of her hand-carved cane, while the other gripped a grocery sack.

"How are you seeing with your new glasses?" I asked.

Mrs. Pennington gave me a grin and moved on into the room.

Her daughter whispered in my ear, "Mother's seeing."

Mrs. Pennington was born and raised on the family farm and had spent eighty-six years there. Only after suffering a broken hip two years ago had she agreed to move in with her daughter in Dallas. Even then, she didn't give up her old ways, rejecting television for the family radio. Her husband had long since died; his tractor had flipped one late fall afternoon and he'd broken his back. She had never learned to drive. What she had needed, she'd picked up on her monthly trek with her husband to Maypearl, a small farming community about fifteen miles west of Waxahachie. After her husband's death, the neighbors continued to help out.

Mrs. Pennington, who'd given birth to her two children at home, had never seen the inside of a hospital or a doctor's office until she broke her hip. I remember her daughter telling me that the only reason her mother had agreed to come for a doctor's visit was that she could no longer read her Bible. My examination revealed that she had dense cataracts. If she wanted to read again, her only option was surgery. When I first suggested it, she balked.

Several months later, I received a call from her daughter. Mrs. Pennington had decided to have the operation, but only on one eye and with several stipulations. First, she rejected the option of an intraocular lens implant in favor of the thick glasses. According to her, the good Lord didn't intend her to have plastic sewn inside her eye. Second, I had to perform the surgery myself. This was because my father was the doctor who had tried to save her husband after he was trapped under the tractor.

Once Mrs. Pennington settled into the exam chair, I asked, "Do you like your new glasses?"

She nodded, still clinging tightly to the wrinkled paper sack. Even though we had been through her surgery and follow-ups together, Mrs. Pennington was never much of a conversationalist. She usually gave only a short reply or gesture.

I performed a brief examination and then slid back on my stool. "Looks like your surgery turned out well."

She thrust the wrinkled sack at me. "I made it for you."

I reached inside and pulled out a crocheted pillow. It was a mixture of dull brown, orange, and faded yellow. The pattern was rife with oversized gaps and missing loops.

"This is very nice," I said.

"It's a seat cushion," she said. "I haven't knitted a thing in over ten years, because I couldn't see. When I got my glasses, I wanted to make you something. You gave me back my sight."

I accepted the compliment, but it wasn't only me Mrs. Pennington was thanking. It was people like Phil, who worked so hard to increase awareness of organ transplantation, and the mortuary students I had just taught to retrieve the tissue. Just as in my early days with Willie, transporting patients around the hospital in Waxahachie, we were all part of an extended team. Suddenly, the oddly shaped pillow took on a whole new meaning. Cradling the cushion in my hands, I knew now that I would find a special place for her gift.

26

PHIL'S SECOND CHANCE

From the start, I could tell Margaret Clark had more on her mind than getting a change of glasses. Margaret Clark was a talker, and listening to her stories and family anecdotes was a part of each visit. I'd grown to understand that listening was an unwritten element of my job description, an aspect of the job you'd think would be appallingly easy. It wasn't. Not when I was busy. Not when I had a waiting room full of patients. On days like today, the time I spent listening would throw my schedule even further behind. Nonetheless, that's what I did.

"Did I tell you," Mrs. Clark said, "my husband and I got divorced. It was final two weeks ago."

I had been seeing Mrs. Clark for years. I understood that Mr. Clark's health was failing. Given his poor health, I never considered divorce a possibility. "How long have you two been married?"

"Fifty-three years in March," the ex-Mrs. Clark said. Margaret pulled a crumpled tissue from her purse and dabbed at her nose. "John's a good man, but I just couldn't take care of him by myself. Our kids have moved off to other parts of the country. John and I decided we had no other choice."

"What's his medical condition?"

"God only knows that he tries, but he's lost all strength in his legs. I'm just not strong enough to lift him. Our only choice was a nursing home."

"Why the divorce?"

"We applied for Medicaid. Together, we don't qualify. Apart, we do."

"What about Social Security benefits?"

"It helps, but it isn't much. We'd put away a little over the years. We'd hoped to have something left over for our kids." She clung to her well-worn Bible. "The nursing home bills, the medicines, they would've bled us dry in a year or two. Our house is paid for, but with the upkeep and taxes, we just manage to get by. Some months it's medicines or food. So we filed for Medicaid."

"Medicaid will pay for John's medicines and the nursing home bills?"

"Only if we're broke," she said.

"What about giving your assets to your children for safekeeping?"

"That should have been done a year ago to qualify for Medicaid. But we didn't know." Her voice strained, as she dabbed again at her nose.

"You're telling me the only way to afford to put John in the nursing home was to get divorced?"

She held up the tattered Bible, its pages frayed from years of use. "All my life, I have lived by what's in here. I've been searching for the answer to how the government can put an end to something God joined together over fifty years ago, and I haven't found it yet."

"Is there anything I can do to help?"

"I could use a prescription for eye drops." Her voice choked with emotion. "Make it out to Margaret Walker. I've taken back my maiden name so the computers at Medicaid don't get confused."

How had we allowed a system that was established to protect those in the greatest need to tear apart our most sacred relationship? On my drive home from work, I passed the pharmacy near my house. Margaret was climbing into her car with her prescription in hand. I waved, but I don't think she saw me.

I was angry at the injustices she had to endure. I'd been angry a lot lately: Angry at Lane Bradley and others who failed to act in their patients' best interests. Angry at insurance companies who forced the Mary Potters of the world to change doctors. I was also angry with myself—I and others who sat around griping about losing control of our profession, while we waited for someone else to fix a system we had at least partially created.

——— ◼ ◼ ———

While I was brooding about injustice and dishonest doctors and America's worsening social service systems, people like Dr. Phil Green were changing the world one day at a time.

In June, Phil asked Janet and me to co-host his donor family at his installation as president of the Texas Medical Association. Phil and his donated liver had made an incredible journey over the last four years. His breakthrough was nothing short of a miracle. Equally miraculous was his list of accomplishments since the liver transplant: He had made several trips to Mexico to deliver humanitarian aid to a remote mountain village. He had established an annual golf tournament to raise money for transplant patients waiting for their second chance at life. He also counseled patients about the unknowns of their life-threatening illnesses.

As TMA president, his newest project was to establish a comprehensive organ-donation awareness program.

"If we can make the program work in Texas," he said, "we'll take it to the American Medical Association and encourage them to copy it across the country."

His enthusiasm was infectious.

That afternoon, Janet and I greeted the donor's parents, Mr. and Mrs. Diaz, at our table in the Hilton Hotel's banquet hall. Uneasy, I took up my assigned seat next to Mrs. Diaz. Janet, always a good conversationalist, introduced us around the table as we exchanged the usual pleasantries. For the next thirty minutes, we made our way through a bland meal, avoiding any talk of their daughter, Susan, or of the event that had brought us all together.

Then Phil stepped up to the lectern.

"I now celebrate two birthdays a year," he said. "One for the day I was born and one for the day I got my new liver from Susan's family."

I was afraid to look at Mr. and Mrs. Diaz.

"I wouldn't be here if it weren't for my donor family." He pointed to our table. An awkward applause rumbled throughout the audience.

"They turned their tragedy into a gift."

Tears filled my eyes. I cast a quick glance in their direction. Their apparent indifference during the first part of the meal was now gone. Phil's heart-wrenching declaration had weakened their stoicism. Janet jammed a tissue in my hand, but I was too embarrassed to use it. I felt the audience's collective joy over Phil's accomplishment collide with the sorrow these parents must have felt with the loss of their daughter.

Phil chronicled events in his life he wouldn't have been alive to enjoy if not for Susan's liver. He spoke of personal triumphs, of family, of work. He extolled the importance of organ transplantation awareness.

"You and I, working together, can make a difference. No one should die without getting a second chance. No one."

My composure vanished as Phil stepped off the dais. There were giants in medicine, people I respected and looked up to. Phil was one of them. I turned to Susan's mother still seated at the table. I wanted to tell her that a part of her daughter lived on, allowing Phil not just to survive, but to help countless others.

Susan's mother's eyes were dry.

She gently laid her hand on my arm. "I cried all my tears when my daughter died. At first, I was angry, but you do what you've got to do to get by." She looked over at Phil who was surrounded by a crowd of well-wishers. "I am thankful that good came from it."

Mrs. Diaz had done something that others and I were reluctant to do—turn her anger into change. Agreeing to donate her daughter's liver had been an action born out of a tragic moment. It wasn't premeditated. It wasn't planned. Her action was her way of making sense of her daughter's death. Not only did her efforts help bring closure to her own grief, but she had begun a chain reaction of goodwill. From her to Phil. From Phil to others.

27

DID I BECOME A BETTER DOCTOR?

The gnawing pain in the pit of my stomach had gotten worse all day. I'd thought it might be gastroenteritis. But without the usual symptoms of nausea and diarrhea, I abandoned that diagnosis and decided I had acute prostatitis. About three in the afternoon, I realized I was in trouble. Unfortunately, there were still two LASIK patients waiting for me before my day was through. By the time I arrived home, I was spent. I'd worn a façade of wellness all day, but now that I was home, I couldn't keep it up any longer.

"I'm sick," I told Janet.

"Did you call Dr. Welton?"

"I didn't want to bother him."

Despite my protests, Janet placed the call. When the call was returned by an associate covering for Dr. Welton, she handed me the receiver. Together, the doctor and I agreed prostatitis was a likely diagnosis, especially since I had suffered a bout several years earlier. She would call in a prescription for a round of antibiotics until I could see Welton in the morning. I agreed, halfheartedly, that if my problem worsened during the night, Janet would bring me to the emergency room. Although I hadn't let Janet in on my plan, I was determined to ride my suffering out until morning when I could go to Welton's office. And maybe I'd get better. I reluctantly put in a call to Babs, asking her to come in early and cancel my morning patients.

Welton's call roused me at just after eight a.m. I really hadn't slept much; intermittent chills had left me wasted but wide awake.

"I think I'm better," I told Welton.

"Just the same, I think you need to come in and let me run a few tests."

The first battery of tests was inconclusive. By then, the antibiotics had begun to kick in. I felt better and considered trying to see my afternoon patients.

Welton said, "We need to do an X-ray of your abdomen. If everything checks out, you can recover at home."

I had almost finished changing back into my street clothes when Welton tapped on the door to the small day surgery room. He wasn't alone.

"You know John Minter?" Welton said. He moved closer to the bed with an X-ray in his hand.

Minter was a general surgeon. That meant the results of my test were not good.

"It looks like you won't be going home quite yet." Welton held up the X-ray. "You have air under your diaphragm."

"What does that mean?" I asked.

Minter stepped forward. "It could be one of three things: First, it could be a ruptured appendix. If that is the case, we'll go in through several small laparoscopy incisions and take it out. It could be a perforated ulcer. I see from the chart that you take a fair amount of Advil, which could be a contributing factor. In that situation, we're usually able to close off the ulcer through small incisions. Either way, you should be able to go home tomorrow and be back to work by the end of the week."

"And the third possibility."

"Let's cross that bridge when we come to it."

I wasn't satisfied, and Minter knew it.

"Option three is a ruptured bowel, probably your colon. The fix is a temporary colostomy."

The third option, if I had it, meant I had diverticulitis—small out-pouchings called tics in the lower portion of the large intestine that can become inflamed and sometimes perforate. I agreed with Minter that option three was a remote possibility.

We were wrong.

When I awoke from surgery, instead of two small Band-aids, I saw a large dressing that extended from my navel down to my pubis. On my left, affixed to my belly, was a plastic bag about the size of my hand—a colostomy pouch to hold my feces. It wasn't until the following day, after I came out of my anesthetic stupor, that I understood what had happened.

I'd had option three: diverticulitis.

The good news was that I didn't have cancer. The bad news was that I'd have to live with a colostomy for three months and then go through the surgery again to put my damaged bowel back together. I was frustrated, maybe even a little angry that I had been dealt this setback. But by the end of the day, I'd decided to count my blessings. It could have been worse. My grandfather had died days after discovering he had colon cancer.

My week's stay in the hospital opened my eyes.

First, I realized that a patient has more to do with the recovery than I ever imagined. Think sick and you feel sick. I remember the moment I decided to get better. Still too weak to step into the shower, I got out my clippers and trimmed my fingernails. It was a small gesture, but a start nonetheless. Second, I discovered that doctors don't get better treatment than anyone else; maybe better communication, but not better treatment. Third, I learned that a word of encouragement from a nurse, aide, or even an orderly went a long way toward lessening my pain and uncertainty.

———— ■ ————

Knowing that everyone would stare, I felt a great deal of trepidation as I returned to the office. That first week, Janet came along to make sure I didn't overdo it. I was determined to look and act normal, even though I was still too sore for street clothes and resorted to wearing scrubs.

My very first patient was Luther Thomas.

"I thought doctors didn't get sick," Luther Thomas said. His eyes moved up and down, appraising me over from head to toe.

"I guess I let my guard down. The chart says you're having trouble seeing the golf ball."

"You play golf, Doc?" Luther asked. "I bet your surgery really slowed you down. What'd you have? Cancer?"

"A ruptured bowel."

Luther must have felt if I could ask medical questions of him, he could do the same of me.

I said, "My doctor told me, except for giving up nuts and popcorn, I should be back to normal soon."

"I think my sister had the same thing you did, Doc. She had one of those bags stuck to her side for the you-know-what to get out. I used to love her cooking, but after that, I just couldn't bring myself to eat anything she made."

Luther's bias was a natural reaction. Since my surgery, I had doubled my time in the shower and still, after his comments, I felt dirty.

"How'd you let it happen, Doc?" He grabbed up his jacket ready to leave. "The rupture of your bowel."

Luther sounded as if he were blaming me, as if doctors had a secret code of immunity.

"They don't know for sure," I said. "Probably something I ate."

My next patient was Eleanor Smart. The most distinctive aspect of Miss Smart's visits was her perfume. Babs claimed she applied it with a paintbrush. I sucked in a breath of fresh air and entered the adjacent exam room.

"Doctor, you've been in my prayers." Eleanor said. She held out her hand to greet me. Her tightly fitting dress revealed little bulges of fat and creases where there shouldn't be. "My nurse friend at the hospital told me all about your surgery. I don't know what I would have done without you."

Eleanor's concern seemed genuine. I was comforted to know that she cared about my well-being. Less comforting was the openness with which my medical problems were discussed by staff at the hospital. The government had recently enacted strict guidelines concerning patient privacy and access to medical records. If my case was any indication, doctors' medical problems were exempt.

"I'll bet you don't know this," Eleanor said, "but I went through the same thing. About two years ago this coming March. My bowel movements hadn't been right for weeks, but I hadn't thought much about it until the pain hit me here below my navel."

Without any prodding, Eleanor gave me a full description of her problems.

Almost in mid-sentence, I interrupted her and said, "When you get sick, it can affect your vision. After you get better, the problems frequently go away. How are your eyes now?"

"I can't read the small print in the newspaper."

I had been able to shift our conversation from bowels to eyes, and now we could get on with the reason for her visit. If there was any consolation in my recent surgery, it was that others had faced similar problems and lived to tell about them. Nevertheless, with an office full of patients, I didn't have time to hear them all.

Having been sick, I was now a better doctor. That was a sentiment I'd heard many times since my surgery. I'm not sure it's true. I'm more understanding, maybe, having suffered through the experience. I'm definitely more sympathetic having received a clearer picture of the role physicians could and should play. I learned not to get defensive when the Luther Thomases raise uncomfortable questions. Not to brush off the Eleanor Smarts when they get sidetracked. If a patient has concerns, then, as their physician, I'm there to help, and if not to help, then to listen.

My father once told me that physicians should view the world through the patients' eyes—not only care for their patients' maladies, but also lead them back up the mountain of their recovery. My experience allowed me an opportunity to take stock of my own practice. To my surprise, I found I was not irreplaceable. The office didn't collapse when I was out convalescing. Granted, my cash flow took a nosedive, but the patients were well taken care of by other physicians. When I returned to work, most of the patients came back. The number of physicians who offered to help was gratifying, indicating that I was indeed part of a medical community.

I also learned that I had obligations to my patients, my family, and to myself. My grandfather had golf; my father his professional organizations. For me, time for myself meant turning the surgical part of my practice over to a younger associate and closing the office down two half-days a month. These were not monumental changes, but enough to spend more time with the people I loved. Ultimately, these less tangible things—understanding, sympathy, becoming a better listener, and spending more time away from the office—made me a better doctor.

EPILOGUE

A lthough I get back to Waxahachie several times a year, I rarely visit the old hospital. In fact, after several renovations and expansions, the red-brick edifice my grandfather helped build in 1921 is barely recognizable today. Ten years ago, I returned for the dedication of a new hospital wing named in honor of my grandfather and father. A year earlier, Baylor Hospital purchased the property and changed the hospital name to Baylor Medical Center at Waxahachie.

Regardless of the name, my family's legacy wasn't in the brick and mortar but in the countless patients throughout Ellis County who were helped by my grandfather, my father, and the institution they supported for more than forty years.

Through three generations of physicians, I've been a witness to an evolution in health care. Many of these changes have led to a widening disparity between the art and the science of medicine, a disparity I hope will someday find an equilibrium.

After the dedication ceremony, I broke free from my hosts and strolled over to the second floor of the original structure, where my grandfather's and father's offices had once been. I was able to find an area that looked vaguely familiar: the waiting room adjacent to my grandfather's office. From there, I stepped inside, closed the door, and moved over to what would have been my grandfather's old office door, the door to a room I had entered hundreds of times. I put my ear to the door. I can't explain the gesture, only that it came naturally and I did it without hesitation.

It's possible I was listening for an echo of long-forgotten conversations. I choose to emulate my father and grandfather, but not to copy them. Their spirits are always with me. Collectively, they serve as a guidepost to mark the course we vowed to follow when each of us took the Hippocratic Oath.

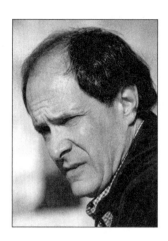

ABOUT THE AUTHOR

R ob Tenery, MD is the third in three generations of physicians whose careers span the last one hundred years. Rob, an ophthalmologist, first began his writing career when he authored commentaries dealing with current events that were impacting the health care profession. His expertise acquired from representing medical organizations on a local, state, and national level led him to becoming a monthly contributor to the nationally distributed periodical, American Medical News, from 1990–1998. It was toward the end of his tenure that he decided to put down on paper a more comprehensive look at the evolution of his chosen profession.

In practice for the last thirty-four years, Rob points out the relevance of the lessons he learned while trailing his grandfather and father during his youth. His compelling stories remind the reader that even a century after his grandfather first set out on horseback to care for the sick and injured with only a small bag of potions and a caring heart, there is still one constant–the patient in need.

Married to his high school sweetheart since 1964, Rob and Janet have two children and four grandchildren. When he is not caring for his patients or lecturing at the University of Texas Southwestern Medical Center at Dallas, their family enjoys relaxing in Santa Fe, New Mexico, where Janet continues her passion of photography and interior design. Rob has taken up hiking in the nearby mountains and working on his next book.